D0955398

Nurses' Aids Series

ARITHMETIC IN NURSING

NURSES' AIDS SERIES

ANAESTHETICS FOR NURSES

ANATOMY AND PHYSIOLOGY FOR NURSES

ARITHMETIC IN NURSING

EAR, NOSE AND THROAT NURSING

MEDICAL NURSING

MICROBIOLOGY FOR NURSES

OBSTETRIC AND GYNAECOLOGICAL NURSING

ORTHOPAEDICS FOR NURSES

PAEDIATRIC NURSING

PERSONAL AND COMMUNITY HEALTH

PHARMACOLOGY FOR NURSES

PRACTICAL NURSING

PRACTICAL PROCEDURES

PSYCHIATRIC NURSING

PSYCHOLOGY FOR NURSES

SURGICAL NURSING

THEATRE TECHNIQUE

TROPICAL HYGIENE AND NURSING

Nurses' Aids Series

Arithmetic in nursing

BY

William C. Fream

S.R.N., B.T.A.Cert.(Hons.)

Senior Tutor, Ballarat Base Hospital, Australia; formerly Senior Tutor Northern Nigeria, and Tutor in Sole Charge, Highwood Hospital for Children, Brentwood, Essex

REVISED BY

R. P. Davies

R.M.N., S.R.N., R.N.T., A.H.A.

Senior Inspector of Training Schools, General Nursing Council for England and Wales

FOURTH EDITION

BAILLIÈRE TINDALL · LONDON

© 1972 BAILLIÈRE TINDALL
7 & 8 Henrietta Street, London W.C.2

A division of Crowell Collier and Macmillan Publishers Ltd

First published August 1956
Reprinted April 1957
Third edition June 1964, 1968
Fourth edition June 1972

ISBN 0 7020 0434 0 Limp edition
ISBN 0 7020 0441 3 Case edition

Published in the United States of America
by the Williams & Wilkins Company, Baltimore

Made and printed in Great Britain by
William Clowes & Sons, Limited
London, Beccles and Colchester

Preface to the Fourth Edition

THE PURPOSE of this book and the background to the writing of it are well expressed in the extract from the original preface printed on p. vii. With the increasing complexity of the equipment that the nurse today may be called upon to handle, the need for a book of this kind is greater than ever.

Arithmetic in Nursing has therefore been considerably revised in this edition in order to help the student with new problems that have arisen. Some old problems cause less difficulty today, but they cannot yet be overlooked in a book of this kind. For instance in the eight years since the last edition there has been a marked increase in the amount of dispensing for individual patients and in the issue of single dose containers. This has led to a decrease in the complexity of calculations which a nurse is required to undertake when administering drugs. It is still essential, however, that she understands the arithmetic that is involved when handling drugs and a number of exercises involving dosage have therefore been retained.

Metrication is well under way and a detailed knowledge of Apothecaries' weights and measures is no longer necessary. Because of this, the chapter on Apothecaries', Avoirdupois and domestic measurements has been omitted. However, measures such as pints and pounds may well continue to be used for a few years and conversion tables and exercises have been included again in this edition. Conversion tables for grains and minims are less likely to be used now, but have been included in an Appendix.

The introduction of decimal currency in 1971 made desirable a special chapter on this topic. It was also thought that a chapter on the uses of statistics and the methods of expressing them (in graphs, histograms, etc.) would be useful, as a prelude, to a deeper study of the subject before going on a management course. Another addition is the new chapter on binary numbers which has been added to enable nurses using computers to gain a little insight into the ways in which computers work.

May 1972   R. P. DAVIES

From the Preface to the First Edition

DURING the last two decades there has been a decided change in many of the features of the art of nursing. The older generation of nurses are wont to complain that proper bedside nursing is slipping away and that the modern nurse is incomplete unless she has a syringe always near at hand. I think they exaggerate a little, because the basic techniques remain the same and always will do so. But they are right to the extent that never before have drugs been given so extensively by subcutaneous, intramuscular and intravenous routes; never before has there been such an array of specialized equipment; and never before has the nurse been expected to delve so deeply into physics, chemistry and mathematics in order to understand the whys and wherefores of all the varieties of treatment now available.

A nurse is required to have a sound grasp of ordinary arithmetic so that such things as calorie requirements, drug dilutions, temperature scales, and metric measurements are something more than a jumble of unmeaning figures. Unfortunately, many a nurse progresses far along the twisting road of training before her mentors become aware of the fact that she lacks a knowledge of basic arithmetic. If such a nurse is to be adequately trained, the tutor has to devote time, that she can ill afford on instruction in subjects that should have been a part of the nurse's mental equipment long before she entered a School of Nursing. What makes the task more difficult is that the degree of knowledge is not uniform, and time usefully spent with one student in bringing her up to standard is time wasted for another who is more advanced.

I have talked to many tutors on this subject and feel that

such a book as this one, which can be placed in the hands of a student and which she can use when alone, will greatly relieve the tutors' anxieties. Those who have become State Registered and are hazy in arithmetic may also find it of assistance, not only in their everyday work, but in enabling them to help the students that are in their charge in the wards.

The chapters are so arranged that instruction in and practice of basic arithmetic techniques are dealt with first. The later chapters apply these techniques to some of the problems constantly met with during the day-to-day work in the wards. It would be a mistake for anyone using this book to think that the early chapters are meant only for those who have no arithmetic. They are meant as a refresher for all those who have left behind their schooldays some years ago, thinking perhaps that they would never need to use a knowledge of arithmetic in their daily work.

Contents

	Preface	v
1	Numbers, prime numbers and factors	1
2	Roman numerals	8
3	Fractions—what they are	11
4	Addition and subtraction of fractions	22
5	Multiplication of fractions	30
6	Division of fractions	35
7	Decimal fractions	38
8	Decimal currency	50
9	The metric system	58
10	Percentages	73
11	Arithmetic and the body fluids	79
12	Solutions	91
13	Dilution of drugs and lotions	104
14	Thermometry	112
15	Heat and calories	127
16	Pressure and its effects	139
17	Graphs	151
18	Uses of statistics	168
19	Computers and the binary number system	190
	Appendix: Useful tables	196
	Answers to questions	205

1
Numbers, prime numbers and factors

FOR CONVENIENCE the human race attaches labels to all things. That in itself makes communication possible. For example, when a person says 'book' everyone has some idea what he means. People in different occupations are likely to conjure up mental images of very different types of book, so we qualify 'book' with adjectives to restrict its meaning, e.g. a ward report book. Thus a clear meaning is conveyed. Such convention is satisfactory until we wish to speak of cost and quantity. Then special adjectives, the numbers, are employed. These are as fundamental to our civilization as speech. Without them any sort of progress in commercial, scientific or social matters would be impossible.

A nurse uses numbers throughout the day. Bed states, estimating the need for and ordering of supplies, giving medicines and keeping charts of various types all require the nurse to be proficient in the use of numbers. Provided the rules are clearly understood and followed the manipulation of numbers is not difficult. The risk of error is reduced if the objects to which numbers refer are always borne in mind when making calculations.

The rules for dealing with problems consisting solely of addition and subtraction, or division and multiplication will be familiar to men and women entering the nursing profession, but it would be wise at this stage to revise the procedure for handling mixed calculations. Sums consisting only of addition and subtraction can be performed in any order without the final result being altered.

Example:

$$24 - 12 + 3 - 2 + 9 - 6 = 12 + 1 + 3 = \textbf{16}$$

similarly

$$24 + 3 + 9 - 12 - 2 - 6 = 36 - 20 \qquad = \textbf{16}.$$

However, if the calculation involves addition or subtraction and multiplication or division the order of work is very important if the correct result is to be obtained. The rule is to deal firstly with multiplication and division, secondly with addition and subtraction. There is an exception to this rule. Brackets are often used in calculations and those parts of the sum within brackets must be worked first. Sometimes it helps to put brackets around parts of the sum when dealing with multiplication and division.

Example 1: Consider the following expression

$$6 \times 12 + 216 \div 3$$

using brackets this equals

$$(6 \times 12) + (216 \div 3)$$
$$= 72 + 72$$
$$= \textbf{144}.$$

If the calculation had been performed in the order in which it was written there would have been an error of 48; a considerable difference. Brackets need not necessarily be inserted in this way once observance of the rule about the precedence of signs becomes habit.

When removing brackets in calculations involving addition and subtraction the rule of signs must be remembered, viz. if the sum within brackets is preceded by a positive sign the signs within the brackets remain unchanged. If a negative sign precedes the bracket, the signs within the bracket must be reversed when the brackets are removed.

Example 2:

Resolve the following expression

$$42 + 7 - (16 - 3) + 7 - (2 - 1)$$

the sums within the brackets can be worked first, i.e.

$$42 + 7 - 13 + 7 - 1$$
$$= 56 - 14$$
$$= \mathbf{42}.$$

alternatively the brackets can be removed

$$42 + 7 - 16 + 3 + 7 - 2 + 1$$
$$= 60 - 18$$
$$= \mathbf{42}.$$

Before leaving the subject of brackets we should remember that two sets of brackets side by side mean that the product of the first set is multiplied by the product of the second set, thus:

$$(2 + 4)(9 - 3) = (6)(6) = \mathbf{36}.$$

From the rule of signs we can see that the product of two positive numbers or two negative numbers is a positive number, and that the product of a positive and a negative number is a negative number.

Example 3:

$$(-6)(+6) = \mathbf{-36}$$
$$(-6)(-6) = \mathbf{+36}$$

Exercises

Now try these:

1. Of 240 patients 120 are visited at the week-end, 80 are visited mid-week, but 40 of these patients are visited at the week-end and mid-week. How many patients received no visitors?

2. $4 + 7 - (7 - 6) + 3 + (4 - 1) = \qquad ?$

3. $7 \times 3 + 27 \div 9 - 3 = \qquad ?$

4. $18 + 27 \times (12 - 9) - 90 = \qquad ?$

5. $(7 + 6)(6 - 3) = \qquad ?$

6. $(-6)(5 - 8) = \qquad ?$

7. $90 \div (3 \times 5) = \qquad ?$

Some numbers are seen to be the product of other, smaller

numbers. For instance 4 is the product of 2×2, 8 is the product of $2 \times 2 \times 2$, six is the product of 2×3 and so on. These smaller numbers are called **factors** of the larger number. Obviously, any number has factors consisting of itself and 1, e.g. $17 = 17 \times 1$, $23 = 23 \times 1$, etc., but these do not count as factors really. Numbers that have only themselves and 1 as factors are called **prime numbers** and it is important to be able to recognize them at sight. The smaller ones are easily recognized. They are 2, 3, 5, 7, 11, 13, 17 and 19. To recognize them when searching for factors of a number saves a great deal of fruitless search.

Factors which are prime numbers are called **prime factors** and, as will be seen in the chapter on addition and subtraction of fractions, finding prime factors is an important process.

Factors of 420 are 42 and 10, but as both these numbers have factors of their own, neither of them are *prime* factors of 420. 10 is the product of 2 and 5 both of which are prime numbers, and 42 is the product of 6 and 7. 7 is a prime number but 6 is the product of two more: 2 and 3. The prime factors of 420 are 2 and 5, 2, 3 and 7. Arranging these in size order we can say that $420 = 2 \times 2 \times 3 \times 5 \times 7$. No amount of dividing will reduce these primes to any other factors.

The prime numbers up to 19 have already been stated above. There are many more, indeed, some mathematicians have spent years extending the list. Their work involves attempting to divide a number by all the known primes, and this involves long division as there is no short method. As far as nursing is concerned, only the smaller ones are likely to be of use. It will be noticed that 1 is not included in the list of prime numbers. Unity is in a special category all its own. Further it will be noticed that 2 is the only even number in the list. A moment's thought will reveal why this is so. All other even numbers are divisible by 2. In other words, 2 is a factor of all even numbers hence they cannot be primes.

Finding the factors of a number involves dividing the number by successive primes starting with 2. To make this task easier there are tests to which the number can be subjected. These are called the 'tests of divisibility'.

Division by 2. All even numbers are divisible by 2, so it can be stated that if the *last* integer of a number is divisible by 2, so is the whole number.

Division by 3. If the sum of the individual integers is divisible by 3, so is the whole number. For example, to discover if the number 241,842 is divisible by 3: Add the individual integers— $2 + 4 + 1 + 8 + 4 + 2 = 21$. As 21 is divisible by 3, so is the big number. $241,842 \div 3 = 80,614$.

Division by 4. If the *last two* integers in a number are divisible by 4, so is the whole number.

Division by 5. Only numbers ending in 0 and 5 are divisible by 5.

Division by 6. All *even* numbers are divisible by 6 if the sum of their integers is divisible by 3. This test is compounded from the test for 2 and for 3, which are the factors of 6.

Division by 7. There is no test for 7 and the only way to determine if it is divisible is to divide by 7 in full.

Division by 8. If the *last three* integers in a number are divisible by 8, so is the whole number.

Division by 9. If the sum of the integers is divisible by 9 so is the whole number. This is similar to the test for 3.

Division by 10. Only numbers ending in 0 are divisible by 10.

Division by 11. This is rather an unusual test. The *alternate* integers are added together. The remaining integers are then added together. This of course results in two numbers. If they are equal, or if their difference is 11 the whole number is divisible by 11.

For example, test to see if 13,937 is divisible by 11.

Add alternate integers: $1 + 9 + 7 = 17$
Add remaining integers: $3 + 3 = 6$
The difference between these: $17 - 6 = 11$

Therefore the number is divisible by 11.

$$11)\overline{13,937}$$
$$\underline{1267}$$

Again: Is 897,437,211 divisible by 11?

$$9 + 4 + 7 + 1 = 21$$
$$8 + 7 + 3 + 2 + 1 = 21$$

The additions are equal, therefore the number is divisible by 11.

$$\frac{11)897,437,211}{81,585,201}$$

These tests are applied to a number to determine its factors. Each test is applied in turn until the number is shown to be divisible by one of the primes. The number is then divided by this prime number and the resulting quotient is tested again until another prime is discovered to divide. The division is carried out and the new quotient is again tested. This is repeated until the last quotient is itself a prime number. The prime numbers are then lined up and these are the prime factors of the number.

Example 1: What are the factors of 112?

(112 is an even number, therefore 2 is a factor)
$112 = 2 \times 56$ (56 is even, so 2 occurs again as a factor)
$ 56 = 2 \times 28$ (28 is even, so 2 occurs yet again as a factor)
$ 28 = 2 \times 14$ (14 is even, so 2 is a factor yet again)
$ 14 = 2 \times 7$ (7 is a prime number, so factors are now complete)
$$112 = 2 \times 2 \times 2 \times 2 \times 7$$

Example 2: What are the prime factors of 150? (150 is even, therefore 2 is a factor)

$150 = 2 \times 75$ (75 is odd, therefore 2 does not occur again as a factor. Test for 3: $7 + 5 = 12$. 12 is divisible by 3 so 75 must be)
$ 75 = 3 \times 25$ (25 is the product of 5 and 5, both of which are prime factors)
$ 25 = 5 \times 5$
$$150 = 2 \times 3 \times 5 \times 5$$

Example 3: Find the factors of 5775. (An odd number

therefore 2 is not a factor. Test for 3: $5 + 7 + 7 + 5 = 24$, which is divisible by 3)

$5775 = 3 \times 1925$ (1925. $1 + 9 + 2 + 5 = 17$. Not divisible by 3. Test for 5. The number ends in 5, so is divisible by 5)

$1925 = 5 \times 385$ (and again)

$385 = 5 \times 77$ (77 is the product of 7 and 11, both of which are primes, so the search ends)

$$5775 = 3 \times 5 \times 5 \times 7 \times 11$$

Example 4: Are the following numbers divisible by 11?

        (a) 8,969,994   (b) 35,728

(a) Sum of alternate digits = $8 + 6 + 9 + 4 = 27$

    Sum of remaining digits = $9 + 9 + 9$ = 27

Therefore the number is divisible by 11.

(b) $3 + 7 + 8 = 18$

                   $5 + 2 = 7$

               $18 - 7 = 11$

Therefore the number is divisible by 11.

Exercises

1. Which of the following numbers are primes?

(a) 6   (b) 7   (c) 4   (d) 3   (e) 9   (f) 13

2. Which of the following numbers are divisible by 3?

(a) 14   (b) 27   (c) 195   (d) 296   (e) 4311

(f) 178,465

3. Which of the following numbers are divisible by 11?

(a) 374   (b) 3740   (c) 9244   (d) 42,966

(e) 345,743,782

4. What are the prime factors of the following numbers?

(a) 12   (b) 14   (c) 35   (d) 38   (e) 138

(f) 380   (g) 924   (h) 525

2
Roman numerals

ROMAN numerals were once extensively used in association with the Apothecaries' measurements. Now that the latter are being replaced by Metric measures and Arabic numbers are being used in preference to Latin terms and symbols, the Roman numerals are tending to fall into disuse. However, they may be occasionally encountered so it would be as well for the nurse to be able to understand them.

The Roman system is extremely unwieldy and this may explain why no outstanding Roman mathematicians emerged from an otherwise enterprising nation. It uses alphabetical letters to represent certain numbers. Small letters are generally used in prescription writing but it is not wrong to use capitals. The numbers of the cranial nerves are usually denoted by capital Roman numerals, and capitals are often used for indicating the hours on clocks and watches and for dates inscribed on tombstones and monuments.

The basic letters used up to one hundred are

i	for unity or one,
v	for five,
x	for ten,
l	for fifty,
and c	for one hundred (cf. our modern usage of cwt for one hundredweight).

To complete the intervening numbers four rules are observed:

(1) Smaller or equal numerals written on the right-hand side of the basic numerals are added together. For instance,

ii	is two, i.e. one plus one.
xx	is twenty, ten plus ten.
xxi	is twenty one, i.e. ten plus ten plus one.

                ccc   is three hundred.
                cxv   is one hundred and fifteen

(2)   A smaller number written on the left-hand side of a basic number is substracted from the basic number. For instance,

                iv   is four, i.e. five minus one.
                ix   is nine, i.e. ten minus one.
                xl   is forty, i.e. fifty minus ten.

Not more than one smaller number is subtracted in this manner.

Nine is ten minus one (ix), but eight is five (v) plus three (viii).

Forty is fifty minus ten (xl), but thirty is three tens (xxx).

(3)   When a smaller number is placed between two larger numbers it is subtracted from the sum of the two larger numbers. For instance,

            xiv   is fourteen, i.e. ten (x) plus five which is fifteen,
                    while the one (i) between is subtracted from
                    this total, making it fourteen.

           xxiv   is therefore twenty-four, i.e. ten plus ten plus
                    five minus one.

            lxix   is sixty-nine, i.e. fifty plus ten plus ten minus
                    one.

(4)   Not more than three similar numerals can stand together. For instance forty could be written as xxxx, but this would not be correct because four similar numerals are standing together. The correct way is xl. It should be noted that when a clock is numbered in Roman numerals four is often denoted by iiii. This is conventional but not strictly correct.

Using these four rules and the five basic numerals already mentioned it is possible to write all the numbers from one to 399.

    1   is i. (A dot is usually placed over the stroke to dis-
          tinguish it from 1 which is fifty. Sometimes a line is
          drawn above the stroke and a dot placed over this
          line to make it clearer still—i̇̄.)

    2   is ii or ï̈ or ij

```
 3   is iii or i̇i̇i̇ or iij
 4   is iv
 5   is v
 6   is vi or vj
 7   is vii or vij
 8   is viii or viij
 9   is ix
10   is x
11   is xi or xj
12   is xii or xij
13   is xiii or xiij
14   is xiv, and so on.
```

Fractions have no expression in Roman numerals with the exception of $\frac{1}{2}$. This is written as 'ss' or 'fs' from the Latin 'semis' (a half).

As has already been noted, dates are usually written in capital letters when Roman numerals are used, and D is used for 500 while M is used for 1000.

Therefore 1972 becomes MCMLXXII

Exercises

Express each of the following as Roman numerals:

1. 2	*2.* 8	*3.* 5	*4.* 17	*5.* 21
6. 28	*7.* 30	*8.* 29	*9.* 18	*10.* 36
11. 41	*12.* 40	*13.* 48	*14.* 55	*15.* 59

Express each of the following in ordinary (Arabic) numbers:

16. ii	*17.* iv	*18.* viii	*19.* xl	*20.* lx
21. vii	*22.* xiv	*23.* xxxviii	*24.* xxiv	*25.* xv
26. xlviii	*27.* lxxxviii	*28.* xvi	*29.* li	*30.* xxii

3
Fractions—what they are

THE NUMBERS discussed so far are called natural numbers when referring to specific quantities of whole objects and integers when negative and positive signs are attached. To enable us to deal with quantities less than whole numbers a special set of numbers called vulgar fractions was evolved. These, together with integers are known as the rational numbers.

We mostly take for granted the use of terms such as 'a quarter of a loaf', 'half an hour', or 'three-quarters of a pint'. Such measurements are used frequently without us stopping to think that we are using fractions, things that are part of a whole and tell us what we want to know in a concise and simple way. In hospitals we must be particularly careful to ensure that information is conveyed in a precise and exact manner. A vivid imagination is not needed to realize the un-helpfulness of giving a consultant vague information such as 'this patient has had a bit of morphia' or 'this patient has had deep X-ray treatment for part of an hour.'

Fractions such as one-half, one-quarter, three-quarters, and their numerical expressions $\frac{1}{2}$, $\frac{1}{4}$, $\frac{3}{4}$, are so familiar to one and all that detailed explanation is not needed. We use them in our everyday life when we talk of such things as half a penny, half a pint, or three-quarters of an inch. Indeed, so familiar are they in such a context that the fact that they *are* fractions tends to be forgotten. On such homely examples can be built many of the fundamental facts that have to be mastered before the mystery is taken out of the manipulation of fractions.

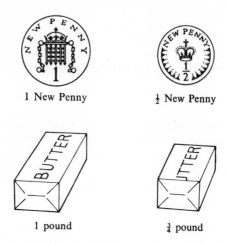

1 New Penny   ½ New Penny

1 pound   ¾ pound

$$\dfrac{3}{4} \begin{array}{l} \to \text{ NUMERATOR} \\ \to \text{ DENOMINATOR} \end{array}$$

Let us examine a fraction, any fraction, and see how it is built up and what information it gives us. ¾ consists of two numbers, set down one over the other with a line between. Three over four. The number under the line is called the **denominator** and tells us that there are four parts to the thing that we happen to be dealing with. The denominator of any fraction will always give us that much information whether it is small as in $\frac{1}{3}$, $\frac{1}{5}$, etc., or whether it is large as in $\frac{1}{1000}$, $\frac{1}{576}$ or $\frac{1}{92}$.

The number above the line is called the **numerator** and it tells us how many of the parts stated in the denominator are being dealt with in that particular instance. Hence in the fraction ¾, something has been divided into four parts and we are dealing with three only of those parts. Similarly in the fraction $\frac{1}{1000}$ there are one thousand parts all told, but only one of them is of immediate concern.

4 parts, therefore
denominator is 4

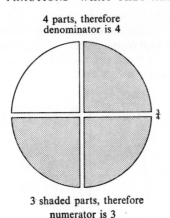

$\frac{3}{4}$

3 shaded parts, therefore
numerator is 3

Now fractions, useful as they are, have their drawbacks, and no one uses them if there is a more understandable way of expressing something. We know that there are 1000 millilitres in a litre, therefore, we usually say that a dose of such and such a medicine is 30 millilitres and not $\frac{3}{100}$ of a litre. It would be perfectly correct to say so and under certain circumstances it might be necessary to say so, but generally speaking we prefer to use whole numbers rather than fractions. Various tables have been devised to avoid fractions. The English systems are somewhat unwieldy and the day is fast approaching when they will pass out of general use in favour of the more rational Metric systems; as they have already with regard to drugs. Until that day arrives we must continue with yards, feet and inches, and pints, fluid ounces and drachms. Only one good thing can be said about such systems, that is, they afford a variety of practice in fractions!

Dividing 1 pint into 20 parts produces 20 fluid ounces, so that 1 fluid ounce can be expressed as $\frac{1}{20}$ of a pint. If we want to express 6 fluid ounces as a fraction of a pint we first say, 'How many fluid ounces are there in a pint ?' There are 20, so that becomes the denominator in the fraction. Next we say, 'How many such parts am I dealing with in this instance ?' 6 such parts, so 6 is the numerator of the fraction, and we can say that 6 fluid ounces is $\frac{6}{20}$ of a pint.

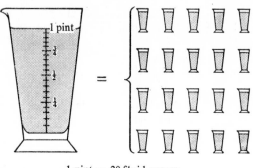

1 pint = 20 fluid ounces
$\frac{1}{20}$ pint = 1 fluid ounce

We go through the same routine if we wish to express inches as a fraction of a foot. There are 12 inches in a foot, therefore 5 inches is $\frac{5}{12}$ of a foot, 11 inches is $\frac{11}{12}$ of a foot and so on.

Before we go any further I would like you to work through some examples. If you fail to achieve full marks or pretty near it you must do one of two things. Either: (a) brush up your tables, or (b) read this section again (or both). You should be able to do most of them mentally.

Exercises

Write as fractions:

1. Nine-sixteenths
2. Two-thirds
3. Three-sevenths
4. Ten-elevenths

Write in words:

5. $\frac{11}{20}$ $\frac{13}{14}$ $\frac{2}{3}$ $\frac{9}{17}$ $\frac{4}{9}$ $\frac{5}{12}$

Express the following as fractions of a pound (weight):

6. 1 ounce
7. 3 ounces
8. 5 ounces
9. 10 ounces
10. 8 ounces
11. 4 ounces

Express the following as fractions of a pound sterling:

12. 5p
13. 25p
14. 30p
15. 75p
16. 80p
17. 60p
18. 35p

Express the following as fractions of a yard:

19. 1 foot
20. 2 feet
21. 3 inches
22. 10 inches

Now try a few the other way round:
Find the values of:

23. $\frac{2}{5}$ of £1
24. $\frac{1}{6}$ of £3
25. $\frac{1}{4}$ of £7
26. $\frac{1}{8}$ of £2
27. $\frac{5}{8}$ of £2
28. $\frac{2}{3}$ of 1 minute
29. $\frac{11}{12}$ of 1 minute
30. $\frac{1}{6}$ of 1 foot
31. $\frac{7}{12}$ of 1 foot
32. $\frac{5}{8}$ of 1 mile
33. $\frac{3}{4}$ of 1 ton

Equivalent Fractions

 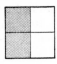 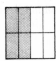 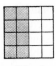

No. 1   No. 2   No. 3   No. 4

Above we have four squares of equal size. The first has been
divided by a line into two halves. The second has been divided
into quarters, the third into eighths, and the last into sixteenths.

Look at the shaded portion in each case and you will see that half the square is shaded, but in No. 2 the shaded portion consists of two quarters, which suggests that the two quarters is the same thing as one half. Similarly, in No. 3, the shaded

8 slices

| 1 half cylinder is 4 slices | $= \frac{4}{8}$ |

Quarter cylinder is 2 slices $= \frac{2}{8}$

Half cylinder is 2 quarters $= \frac{2}{4}$

$$\frac{1}{2} = \frac{2}{4} = \frac{4}{8}$$

portion consists of four eighths, and, yet again, in No. 4, the shaded half consists of eight sixteenths. In other words we can say from this illustration that $\frac{1}{2}$ is the same as $\frac{2}{4}$ or $\frac{4}{8}$ or $\frac{8}{16}$. They are all expressed in different values but they are all equal.

This leads us to a very important principle: The value of a fraction remains unaltered **when the numerator and the denominator are multiplied or divided by the same number.**

Frequently a fraction is some astronomical number that conveys no meaning whatever until it has been reduced to manageable size. For instance $\frac{40}{1000}$ is an unwieldy fraction. If we apply the above principle and divide the numerator by 2 and then the denominator by the same number, 2, the fraction becomes $\frac{20}{500}$ We can repeat the performance again and make the fraction $\frac{10}{250}$ and yet again, making it $\frac{5}{125}$. If we then divide above and below by 5 the fraction is reduced to a form that permits of no further reduction, namely $\frac{1}{25}$

and we can see that $\frac{40}{1000} = \frac{1}{25}$. This process is called reducing the fraction to its lowest terms, and is done by a process called 'cancelling' or 'cancelling out'. For brevity it is usually written as follows:

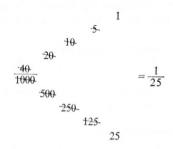

$$= \frac{1}{25}$$

Each division is done mentally and the result each time is entered in smaller figures and at a slightly higher level. Two things are essential when using this method. One is that each division of the numerator is accompanied by a division of the denominator by the same number and the other is that the quotients (results of the division) must be entered neatly or confusion arises.

Cancelling in fractions is more commonly required than expanding, but it is sometimes necessary to multiply. If the following fractions are required to be arranged in increasing order of size, it can be done quite simply by observing the numerators.

$$\frac{6}{20} \qquad \frac{4}{20} \qquad \frac{9}{20} \qquad \frac{13}{20} \qquad \frac{1}{20}$$

The correct order is:

$$\frac{1}{20} \qquad \frac{4}{20} \qquad \frac{6}{20} \qquad \frac{9}{20} \qquad \frac{13}{20}$$

But in the following example

$$\frac{1}{2} \qquad \frac{7}{12} \qquad \frac{1}{3} \qquad \frac{3}{4}$$

it is not obvious at first glance which is greater or lesser than any of the others. It remains obscure until all the fractions are rewritten with the same denominator. 12 is a convenient denominator for this case. To give the fraction $\frac{1}{2}$ a denominator of 12 we must multiply the denominator by 6. If we do this we must also multiply the numerator by 6. In this way $\frac{1}{2}$ becomes $\frac{6}{12}$.

Similarly by multiplying the denominator and numerator of $\frac{1}{3}$ by 4, $\frac{1}{3}$ becomes $\frac{4}{12}$. And by multiplying $\frac{3}{4}$ by 3, it becomes $\frac{9}{12}$.

We can then rewrite the fractions thus:

$$\frac{6}{12} \qquad \frac{7}{12} \qquad \frac{4}{12} \qquad \frac{9}{12}$$

and can then arrange them easily in correct size order

$$\frac{4}{12} \qquad \frac{6}{12} \qquad \frac{7}{12} \qquad \frac{9}{12}$$

which corresponds with

$$\frac{1}{3} \qquad \frac{1}{2} \qquad \frac{7}{12} \qquad \frac{3}{4}$$

Later, when we come to consider the addition and subtraction of fractions, this process of multiplying up with a common denominator is essential.

Exercises

Fill in the gaps left in the following:

1. $\dfrac{1}{2} = \dfrac{5}{?} = \dfrac{7}{?} = \dfrac{?}{22} = \dfrac{?}{40}$

2. $\dfrac{3}{4} = \dfrac{6}{?} = \dfrac{12}{?} = \dfrac{?}{8} = \dfrac{?}{12}$

3. $\dfrac{3}{5} = \dfrac{?}{10} = \dfrac{?}{25} = \dfrac{21}{?} = \dfrac{36}{?}$

4. $\dfrac{5}{8} = \dfrac{15}{?} = \dfrac{30}{?} = \dfrac{?}{16} = \dfrac{?}{72}$

Reduce the following to their lowest terms:

5. $\frac{2}{6}$ 8. $\frac{4}{12}$ 11. $\frac{21}{28}$ 14. $\frac{21}{72}$

6. $\frac{2}{10}$ 9. $\frac{16}{40}$ 12. $\frac{25}{80}$ 15. $\frac{15}{40}$

7. $\frac{3}{9}$ 10. $\frac{28}{35}$ 13. $\frac{13}{52}$ 16. $\frac{14}{91}$

In each of the following pairs, express the first part as a fraction (in the lowest terms) of the second part:

17.	6p; 12p	27.	1 ft; 1 yd
18.	3p; 12p	28.	6 in; 1 ft
19.	6 oz; 1 lb	29.	6 in; 2 ft
20.	12 oz; 1 lb	30.	6 in; 3 ft
21.	7½ milligrams; 30 milligrams	31.	6 in; 1 yd
22.	1½ milligrams; 12 milligrams	32.	½ p; 3 p
		33.	1p; £1
23.	10 millilitres; 1 litre	34.	25p; 100p
24.	5 millilitres; 10 centilitres	35.	25p; 75p
		36.	30 sec; 10 min
		37.	40 min; 1 hr
25.	20 milligrams; 1 gramme	38.	3 qt; 2 gal
26.	2 millilitres; 4 centilitres		

So far the fractions we have dealt with have all been 'proper' fractions. That is to say, that the numerators have all been smaller than the denominators, e.g. $\frac{3}{4}$, $\frac{7}{12}$, $\frac{91}{120}$. There are, however, such things as 'improper' fractions though there is nothing wrong about them. An improper fraction is one in which the numerator is bigger than the denominator, e.g. $\frac{7}{4}$, $\frac{9}{2}$, $\frac{8}{3}$. Let us take the first of these and see what we have.

$\frac{7}{4}$ can be said 'seven-quarters', and if there are seven quarters there is enough to make 1 unit with $\frac{3}{4}$ over. Hence $\frac{7}{4}$ can be written down as $1\frac{3}{4}$.

Similarly, $\frac{5}{2}$ can be spoken of as five halves, and with five halves there is enough to make 2 whole units with $\frac{1}{2}$ over, so that $\frac{5}{2}$ can be written as $2\frac{1}{2}$.

Then again, $\frac{8}{3}$ is eight-thirds which makes 2 whole units and $\frac{2}{3}$ over, so that $\frac{8}{3}$ can be expressed as $2\frac{2}{3}$.

Numbers that consist partly of a whole number and partly of a fraction are called mixed numbers.

From this it follows that to rewrite an improper fraction as a mixed number it is necessary to divide the numerator by the

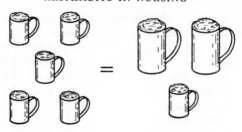

5 half-litres = 2½ litres

denominator putting down the quotient (result of the division) as a whole number and the remainder as the fraction part.

Exercises

Try a few:

Express the following improper fractions as mixed numbers:

1. $\frac{5}{2}$	*4.* $\frac{8}{5}$	*7.* $\frac{29}{11}$	*9.* $\frac{28}{12}$
2. $\frac{5}{4}$	*5.* $\frac{11}{4}$	*8.* $\frac{18}{7}$	*10.* $\frac{32}{9}$
3. $\frac{7}{3}$	*6.* $\frac{48}{8}$		

Conversely when it is necessary to convert mixed numbers into improper fractions, the whole number part is multiplied by the denominator and the numerator is **added** to the product (result of the multiplication).

Like this. Convert $4\frac{1}{4}$ into an improper fraction.

First multiply the whole number, 4, by the denominator, 4, = 16.

Then add the numerator, 1.

$$1 + 16 = 17$$

Therefore the improper fraction is $\frac{17}{4}$

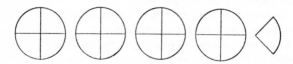

Quarters
$$4 + 4 + 4 + 4 + 1$$
$$= 17 \text{ quarters}$$
$$4\tfrac{1}{4} = \tfrac{17}{4}$$

Exercises

Try these:

Express the following as improper fractions:

1. $1\tfrac{1}{3}$	*4.* $3\tfrac{1}{8}$	*7.* $3\tfrac{7}{10}$	*9.* $9\tfrac{2}{7}$
2. $1\tfrac{2}{3}$	*5.* $4\tfrac{3}{8}$	*8.* $4\tfrac{3}{10}$	*10.* $5\tfrac{17}{100}$
3. $2\tfrac{3}{4}$	*6.* $7\tfrac{1}{8}$		

4

Addition and subtraction of fractions

ADD the following:

6 apples and 3 apples and 7 apples and 2 apples.

The answer is 18 apples, is it not?

Now add these:

6 apples and 3 pears and 7 oranges and 2 melons.

The proper answer is that the sum cannot be done as it stands as these are sets of different things; in other words things with different denominations. In order to do the sum they must all be of the same denomination. We can get round the difficulty by saying that they are all fruits and therefore there are 18 fruits in all.

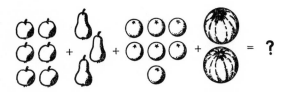

So it is with fractions.

It is easy enough to add $\frac{1}{12}$, $\frac{3}{12}$, $\frac{6}{12}$ and $\frac{7}{12}$, because they all have the same denomination, or denomin*ator* in the case of fractions. The answer is $\frac{17}{12}$ which we can condense to the mixed number $1\frac{5}{12}$.

But when we come to consider the sum of $\frac{1}{12}$, $\frac{1}{4}$, $\frac{1}{2}$ and $\frac{2}{3}$ we meet the same problem as in the apples, pears, oranges

22

and melons. These fractions all have different demoninators and to make any sense out of them we must first provide them with the same denominator.

This involves finding a suitable denominator and, whereas any denominator will do, it is less cumbersome to use the lowest number into which all will divide. In this case 12 is the lowest.

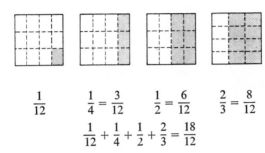

$$\frac{1}{12} \qquad \frac{1}{4} = \frac{3}{12} \qquad \frac{1}{2} = \frac{6}{12} \qquad \frac{2}{3} = \frac{8}{12}$$

$$\frac{1}{12} + \frac{1}{4} + \frac{1}{2} + \frac{2}{3} = \frac{18}{12}$$

First we write down the sum:

$$\tfrac{1}{12} + \tfrac{1}{4} + \tfrac{1}{2} + \tfrac{2}{3}$$

Then we must take each one separately and multiply the denominator so that it is valued at 12 not forgetting that whenever we multiply a denominator we must also multiply the numerator by the same amount.

The first is already in twelfths and needs no changing.

The second, $\frac{1}{4}$, must be multiplied by three above and below and becomes $\frac{3}{12}$.

The third must be multiplied by 6 above and below so that it becomes $\frac{6}{12}$.

And the last by 4 to make it $\frac{8}{12}$.

The sum can then be rewritten thus:

$$\tfrac{1}{12} + \tfrac{3}{12} + \tfrac{6}{12} + \tfrac{8}{12}$$

We can now add it very simply and it is $\frac{18}{12}$, or as a mixed number $1\frac{6}{12}$, which is the same as $1\frac{1}{2}$.

Here are three worked examples showing how: (*a*) an

addition can be set out, (b) how a subtraction can be set out, and (c) how a mixed problem can be set out.

(a) Find the sum of $\frac{1}{2}$, $\frac{5}{6}$, $\frac{2}{3}$, $\frac{2}{5}$. (A suitable denominator is 30.)

$$\frac{1}{2} = \frac{15}{30}$$
$$\frac{5}{6} = \frac{25}{30}$$
$$\frac{2}{3} = \frac{20}{30}$$
$$\frac{2}{5} = \frac{12}{30}$$

$$\therefore \; \frac{1}{2} + \frac{5}{6} + \frac{2}{3} + \frac{2}{5} = \frac{15}{30} + \frac{25}{30} + \frac{20}{30} + \frac{12}{30}$$
$$= \frac{72}{30}$$
$$= 2\frac{12}{30}$$
$$= 2\frac{2}{5}$$

(b) Find the value of $3\frac{1}{5} - 1\frac{2}{15} - \frac{2}{3}$. (15 is a suitable denominator.)

$$= \frac{16}{5} - \frac{17}{15} - \frac{2}{3} \text{ (Converting to improper fractions)}$$
$$\frac{16}{5} = \frac{48}{15}$$
$$\frac{2}{3} = \frac{10}{15}$$
$$= \frac{48 - 17 - 10}{15}$$
$$= \frac{21}{15} = 1\frac{2}{5}$$

(c) Find the value of $4\frac{1}{4} - 2\frac{1}{8} - \frac{3}{4} + 6\frac{2}{3}$

$$= 4\frac{1}{4} + 6\frac{2}{3} - 2\frac{1}{8} - \frac{3}{4} \quad \text{(Re-arranging so that pluses come first and minuses last)}$$
$$= \frac{17}{4} + \frac{20}{3} - \frac{17}{8} - \frac{3}{4} \quad \text{(Converting to improper fractions)}$$

(24 is a convenient common denominator.)

$$\frac{17}{4} = \frac{102}{24}$$
$$\frac{20}{3} = \frac{160}{24}$$
$$\frac{17}{8} = \frac{51}{24}$$
$$\frac{3}{4} = \frac{18}{24}$$
$$= \frac{102 + 160 - 51 - 18}{24}$$
$$= \frac{193}{24} = 8\frac{1}{24}$$

In the examples just worked, a suitable denominator was taken without giving any explanation of how it was derived. As stated previously, any denominator will do so long as it is divisible by all the denominators of the fractions in the sum.

Now a set of numbers can have any number of multiples, e.g. multiples of the numbers 3, 4 and 6 are 12, 24, 36, 48, but the lowest of these is 12. In other words, 12 is the lowest number that is capable of division by 3 and 4 and 6. This is usually called the **lowest common multiple**, or, if we are dealing with the denominators of fractions, the **lowest common denominator**. Where this is not obvious at a glance, there is a special way of discovering it.

To find the lowest common multiple (LCM), of a series of numbers:

(1)   Set down the numbers in decreasing size order.

(2)   Alongside each number write down the factors of that number.

(3)   Underneath, in the next line, take each number in turn and write down all the factors in a line, but leaving out any factors that have occurred in previous numbers unless there are more factors in the number under consideration than appear with any previous number.

(4)   Check to see that all the factors from any number appear in the line.

(5)   Multiply all these factors to find the LCM.

A few worked examples will make this clear.

(*a*)   Find the LCM of the following numbers: 6, 8, 12, 4, 2.

First set down the number in descending size order, i.e. the highest first. Then write the factors alongside.

$$12 = 2 \times 2 \times 3$$
$$8 = 2 \times 2 \times 2$$
$$6 = 2 \times 3$$
$$4 = 2 \times 2$$
$$2 = 2 \times 1$$

Next write the factors from each number in a line omitting any that occur in a previous number unless there are insufficient.

$2 \times 2 \times 3$ (from 12—all its factors), $\times 2$ (from 8 we already have two 2s from 12 so we can omit them from 8 and need only one more). We need take none from 6 as they have occurred already. Similarly none from 4 or from 2.

We are left with $2 \times 2 \times 3 \times 2$. Checking back to make sure we see that we have all the factors of 12, all the factors of 8, all the factors of 6, and 4, and 2 (the 1 does not count).

Multiplying these we get 24. So 24 is the LCM.

(*b*) Find the LCM of 15, 3, 6, 9 and 2.

Size order and factors:

$$15 = 3 \times 5$$
$$9 = 3 \times 3$$
$$6 = 2 \times 3$$
$$3 = 3 \times 1$$
$$2 = 2 \times 1$$

Each number in turn:

$$(3 \times 5)(\times 3)(\times 2)$$

Therefore LCM = 90

(*c*) Find the lowest common **denominator** of

$$\tfrac{1}{10}, \tfrac{1}{4}, \tfrac{1}{8} \text{ and } \tfrac{1}{15}$$

Size order of denominators:

$$15 = 3 \times 5$$
$$10 = 2 \times 5$$
$$8 = 2 \times 2 \times 2$$
$$4 = 2 \times 2$$

Numbers in turn:

$$(3 \times 5)(\times 2)(\times 2 \times 2)$$

Lowest common denominator = 120

Exercises

Here are some involving addition, subtraction and the finding of lowest common denominators:

1. 2 sevenths + 3 sevenths	*6.* $\frac{8}{9} - \frac{2}{9}$
2. 5 ninths + 2 ninths	*7.* $\frac{3}{4} - \frac{1}{4}$
3. $\frac{1}{3} + \frac{5}{9}$	*8.* $\frac{1}{2} + \frac{1}{5}$
4. $\frac{1}{8} + \frac{5}{8}$	*9.* $\frac{1}{3} + \frac{1}{5}$
5. $\frac{2}{9} + \frac{7}{9}$	*10.* $\frac{1}{4} + \frac{3}{5}$

11. $\frac{1}{3} + \frac{1}{6}$ *19.* $\frac{4}{9} + \frac{1}{3} + \frac{5}{6}$

12. $\frac{3}{4} - \frac{2}{3}$ *20.* $\frac{1}{2} + \frac{1}{4} - \frac{3}{8}$

13. $\frac{5}{6} + \frac{2}{9}$ *21.* $\frac{3}{4} - \frac{1}{9} + \frac{1}{3}$

14. $\frac{1}{4} + \frac{5}{8}$ *22.* $\frac{3}{7} - \frac{1}{4} + \frac{1}{14}$

15. $1 - \frac{2}{7}$ *23.* $\frac{2}{3} + \frac{7}{10} - \frac{4}{15}$

16. $3 - \frac{4}{5}$ *24.* $\frac{2}{3} + \frac{1}{7} - \frac{4}{21}$

17. $\frac{7}{8} - \frac{5}{16}$ *25.* $\frac{5}{6} - \frac{17}{25} + \frac{3}{10}$

18. $\frac{3}{5} + \frac{3}{10} + \frac{1}{2}$

When the sums to be done consist of mixed numbers, which you will remember are partly whole numbers and partly fractions, it is best to deal with the whole numbers first and the fraction part separately. Also, where the fraction is an improper one, it is best to convert it to a mixed number before starting.

For example:

(*a*) Simplify $7\frac{3}{4} - 4\frac{1}{3}$

First deal with the whole numbers and rewrite the expression. The fractions can be provided with a common denominator at the same time in this particular example.

$$7 - 4 + \frac{9}{12} - \frac{4}{12}$$
$$= 3 + \frac{5}{12}$$
$$= 3\frac{5}{12}$$

(*b*) Simplify $4 - 1\frac{5}{6} - 2\frac{8}{15} + 5\frac{1}{10}$

Rearrange the expression so that the pluses come first

$$= 4 + 5\frac{1}{10} - 1\frac{5}{6} + 2\frac{8}{15}$$

Next deal with the whole numbers and provide a common denominator for the fractions. This can be discovered in the margin.

$$= 4 + 5 - 1 - 2 + \frac{3}{30} - \frac{25}{30} - \frac{16}{30}$$
$$= 6 + \frac{3 - 25 - 16}{30}$$
$$= 6 - \frac{38}{30}$$
$$= 6 - 1\frac{4}{15}$$
$$= 4\frac{11}{15}$$

$15 = 3 \times 5$
$10 = 2 \times 5$
$6 = 2 \times 3$
$3 \times 5 \times 2 = 30$

(c) $1 - \frac{2}{5} - \frac{2}{9}$ (In this it is best to subtract $\frac{2}{5}$ from 1 leaving only a simple fraction subtraction)

$$= \frac{3}{5} - \frac{2}{9}$$
$$= \frac{27}{45} - \frac{10}{45}$$
$$= \frac{17}{45}$$

Exercises

Simplify:

1. $1\frac{1}{8} + 3\frac{5}{8}$
2. $2\frac{3}{10} + 4\frac{3}{10}$
3. $2\frac{3}{12} - \frac{7}{12}$
4. $1\frac{1}{2} + 3\frac{1}{3}$
5. $2\frac{1}{4} + 5\frac{2}{3}$
6. $3\frac{1}{9} + 4\frac{5}{12}$
7. $5\frac{1}{16} - 2\frac{1}{8}$

8. $11\frac{2}{3} - 3\frac{1}{4}$
9. $3\frac{4}{5} - 3\frac{2}{3}$
10. $4\frac{4}{5} + 3\frac{3}{10} - 6\frac{1}{2}$
11. $5\frac{1}{4} - 3\frac{3}{8} + 1\frac{1}{2}$
12. $2\frac{6}{30} - 2\frac{8}{15} + 4\frac{5}{6} - 3\frac{2}{3}$
13. $11\frac{2}{3} - 3\frac{2}{5} - 2\frac{4}{9} + 1\frac{1}{6}$

All the problems so far have been devised simply as a means of exercising the knowledge gained in the manipulation of fractions. There is a far more interesting way of doing this once the basic skill has been attained and that is by tackling various real life situations. True enough, many of these situations are a little far-fetched but many of them are not. Bear with me in working through the silly ones for the sake of being able to do the real ones.

First an example:

Four patients engaged on industrial therapy are packing electrical equipment into boxes. In 1 hour Mr Jones packed $\frac{3}{4}$ of a box, Mrs Thomas packed $\frac{1}{2}$ a box, Miss Smith packed $\frac{1}{10}$ of a box and Mr Brown packed $\frac{2}{5}$ of a box. What is the total amount packed in an hour?

The amount packed is $\frac{3}{4} + \frac{1}{2} + \frac{2}{5} + \frac{1}{10}$
$$= \frac{15}{20} + \frac{10}{20} + \frac{8}{20} + \frac{2}{20} = \frac{35}{20}$$
$$\frac{35}{20} = 1\frac{3}{4} \text{ boxes in 1 hour.}$$

Exercises

Try a few:

1. The tea tin contained 2 lb tea on Monday. $\frac{1}{4}$ lb was used on Monday, $\frac{7}{16}$ was used on Tuesday, and on Wednesday and Thursday $\frac{3}{8}$ lb each day. How much is left for the rest of the week?

2. £50 is deposited by a relative in an hospital account for a mentally handicapped person. $\frac{1}{4}$ is to be spent on extra clothing; $\frac{3}{10}$ on comic papers; and $\frac{2}{5}$ on fares and shopping in the local town. How much can be spent in the hospital shop?

3. Four part-time nurses are engaged to assist three full-time nurses in an hospital department. Their respective hours of duty add up to the following proportions of a full working week: $\frac{1}{2}$, $\frac{3}{8}$, $\frac{3}{4}$, $\frac{5}{8}$. What is the total equivalent number of full-time nursing staff?

4. There are 40 patients in a ward on Monday morning. $\frac{1}{10}$ are discharged on Tuesday, $\frac{3}{20}$ on Wednesday, $\frac{1}{4}$ on Thursday. If 15 patients were admitted during that time how many empty beds are there?

5. Johnny sends a cake to the kitchen with instructions that $\frac{1}{10}$ is to be given to Mike and $\frac{2}{5}$ to Sam, and he eats $\frac{1}{4}$ himself. How much remains?

6. A leaky pipe drips at the rate of $\frac{1}{2}$ pint an hour. If a bowl is placed under it and contains $2\frac{1}{2}$ quarts when you go on duty, how long will it be before it is full if it will hold $1\frac{1}{2}$ gallons?

7. A new tape recording is being made of a group of patients suffering from speech defects. They speak for $4\frac{1}{2}$, $3\frac{1}{2}$, $4\frac{5}{12}$, and $3\frac{7}{12}$ minutes respectively. How long does the recording last?

5
Multiplication of fractions

WHEN two or more fractions are to be multiplied together the numerators are multiplied together separately from the denominators, and then all the denominators are multiplied. For example, in the expression $\frac{3}{4} \times \frac{1}{2}$, the numerators 3 and 1 are first multiplied giving a product of 3. 3 becomes the new numerator. Next the denominators 4 and 2 are multiplied giving a product of 8. This becomes the new denominator, so that the new fraction is $\frac{3}{8}$.

$$\frac{3}{4} \times \frac{1}{2} = \frac{3 \times 1}{4 \times 2} = \frac{3}{8}$$

A half of three-quarters is three-eighths.

Logically speaking, multiplying by a fraction is an absurdity, because the very word 'multiply' implies that as a result of the multiplication there will be more than there was formerly. Yet, from the forgoing example, it can be seen that as a result of 'multiplying' by $\frac{1}{2}$ there is less than there was originally. If the expression had asked, 'What is $\frac{1}{2}$ of $\frac{3}{4}$?', it would have been both logical and correct. To cover this point mathematicians have arranged a convention, a sort of poetic licence, to regard the word 'of' in such expressions as meaning the same as would a multiplication sign. In this way such problems as the following can be written in mathematical terms.

There are 40 patients in a ward. $\frac{3}{4}$ *of* these are confined to bed but $\frac{2}{3}$ *of* the bed patients are allowed to wash themselves. How many bowls will be required for their use?

Number of bowls required $= 40 \times \frac{3}{4} \times \frac{2}{3}$

$$= \frac{\overset{10}{\cancel{40}} \times \overset{1}{\cancel{3}} \times 2}{\underset{1}{\cancel{4}} \times \underset{1}{\cancel{3}}}$$

$$= \frac{10 \times 1 \times 2}{1 \times 1}$$

$$= 20$$

Where whole numbers are concerned in the multiplication of fractions, they should be regarded as fractions with a denominator of 1. This prevents confusion as to whether a whole number is to be multiplied by the denominator or the numerator, as the rule of multiplying only numerators together, and only denominators together can then be applied. Naturally, providing a denominator of 1 does not alter the value of the whole number as any number divided by 1 remains the same. For instance the number 2 is still valued as two even though it is expressed in fractional form of $\frac{2}{1}$.

Example: Multiply $\frac{3}{5}$ by 2.

$$\frac{3}{5} \times 2 = \frac{3}{5} \times \frac{2}{1} = \frac{3 \times 2}{5 \times 1} = \frac{6}{5} = 1\frac{1}{5}$$

The question—'Why should the numerator of a fraction be multiplied by a whole number? Why not the denominator as well?'—can be answered if one returns to the original explanation of what a fraction is. There it was stated that the denominator tells one how many parts a thing has been divided into, and if the word 'apples' is substituted for 'fifths' in the example above, the expression would read, 'multiply 3 "apples" by 2'. The answer is 6 'apples' just as the answer above was 6 'fifths'.

Cancelling can help to simplify multiplication of fractions a great deal. In the expression—multiply $\frac{5}{12}$ by $\frac{12}{25}$, numerators are going to be multiplied together and so are denominators, arriving at a fraction of $\frac{60}{300}$. This is not in its simplest form, however, and to simplify one would have to divide numerator and denominator first by twelve and then by five, reducing it to $\frac{1}{5}$. How unnecessary it would be to multiply by twelve and then divide by twelve in the next step. Cancelling will solve the problem. Set the work out thus:

$$\frac{5}{12} \times \frac{12}{25} = \frac{5 \times 12}{12 \times 25}$$

Cancelling can then proceed. Twelve in the top line and twelve in the bottom line are both divisible by twelve. Five in the top line and twenty-five in the bottom line are both divisible by five, so the expression will look like this after cancellation:

$$\frac{\overset{1}{\cancel{5}} \times \overset{1}{\cancel{12}}}{\underset{1}{\cancel{12}} \times \underset{5}{\cancel{25}}} = \frac{1 \times 1}{1 \times 5} = \frac{1}{5}$$

Another example: Simplify $\frac{6}{35} \times \frac{14}{15}$

$$= \frac{\overset{2}{\cancel{6}} \times \overset{2}{\cancel{14}}}{\underset{5}{\cancel{35}} \times \underset{5}{\cancel{15}}}$$

(6 in the numerator and 15 in the denominator divisible by 3; 14 and 35 divisible by 7)

$$= \frac{2 \times 2}{5 \times 5} = \frac{4}{25}$$

And again:

Multiply together $\frac{3}{10}$, $\frac{8}{9}$ and $\frac{3}{4}$

$$= \frac{\overset{1}{\cancel{3}} \times \overset{\overset{1}{2}}{\cancel{8}} \times \overset{1}{\cancel{3}}}{\underset{5}{\cancel{10}} \times \underset{3}{\cancel{9}} \times \underset{1}{\cancel{4}}}$$

$$= \frac{1 \times 1 \times 1}{5 \times 1 \times 1} = \frac{1}{5}$$

Exercises

Simplify:

1. $\frac{1}{2} \times \frac{1}{4}$
2. $\frac{3}{4} \times \frac{1}{4}$
3. $\frac{3}{8} \times \frac{2}{3}$
4. $\frac{7}{8} \times 2$
5. $\frac{4}{9} \times 3$
6. $\frac{5}{6} \times \frac{1}{5}$
7. $4 \times \frac{1}{4}$
8. One-third of four-fifths
9. $\frac{3}{7}$ of 4
10. A quarter of 2 litres

In all the above exercises only simple fractions have been used. When the fraction is a mixed number, i.e. partly a whole number and partly fraction as in $2\frac{1}{2}$, it must be converted into an improper fraction before work starts. This is different from questions involving addition and subtraction where, it will be remembered, the whole number parts could be dealt with separately. Hence in the expression $2\frac{1}{2} + 3\frac{3}{4} - 1\frac{3}{8}$, the whole number part resulted in 4, and the fraction parts in $\frac{7}{8}$.

In multiplication the fractions must be rewritten as improper fractions so that using the same fractions the expression is $2\frac{1}{2} \times 3\frac{3}{4} \times 1\frac{3}{8}$. Re-written it becomes

$$\frac{5}{2} \times \frac{15}{4} \times \frac{11}{8}$$

The rule of multiplying numerators together and denominators together can then be used, and it becomes

$$\frac{5 \times 15 \times 11}{2 \times 4 \times 8}$$
$$= \frac{825}{64}$$
$$= 12\frac{57}{64}$$

$$
\begin{array}{r}
12 \\
64)\overline{825} \\
64 \\
\hline
185 \\
128 \\
\hline
57
\end{array}
$$

Here again, cancelling can simplify the working to a considerable extent. In the above expression there were no factors common to both the numerator and the denominator, so no cancelling could be done.

Example 1: Simplify $3\frac{1}{5} \times 3\frac{5}{8} \times 1\frac{6}{29}$

$$\frac{16}{5} \times \frac{29}{8} \times \frac{35}{29}$$

$$= \frac{\overset{2}{16} \times \overset{1}{29} \times \overset{7}{35}}{\underset{1}{5} \times \underset{1}{8} \times \underset{1}{29}}$$

$$= \frac{2 \times 1 \times 7}{1 \times 1 \times 1}$$

$$= \mathbf{14}$$

Cancelling has taken all the extensive multiplying and dividing out of the work. 29 was divisible by 29 in both numerator and denominator. So were 16 by 8 and 35 by 5.

Example 2: Simplify $\frac{3}{4} \times 3\frac{1}{7} \times 1\frac{4}{11} \times \frac{1}{5} \times 7$

$$= \frac{3}{4} \times \frac{22}{7} \times \frac{15}{11} \times \frac{1}{5} \times \frac{7}{1}$$

$$= \frac{3 \times \overset{2}{22} \times \overset{3}{15} \times 1 \times \overset{1}{7}}{\underset{2}{4} \times \underset{1}{7} \times \underset{1}{11} \times \underset{1}{5} \times \underset{1}{1}}$$

$$= \frac{3 \times 1 \times 3 \times 1 \times 1}{2 \times 1 \times 1 \times 1 \times 1}$$

$$= \frac{9}{2}$$

$$= 4\frac{1}{2}$$

Exercises

Simplify:

1. $\frac{2}{7} \times 3$	*8.* $\frac{5}{28} \times 21$	*15.* $3\frac{1}{3} \times 6$
2. $\frac{4}{9} \times 5$	*9.* $\frac{2}{7} \times \frac{3}{5}$	*16.* $4\frac{2}{3} \times 1\frac{1}{5}$
3. $\frac{5}{12} \times 6$	*10.* $\frac{4}{11} \times \frac{3}{8}$	*17.* $9\frac{5}{11} \times \frac{11}{13}$
4. $\frac{7}{8} \times 4$	*11.* $\frac{3}{4}$ of 8	*18.* $2\frac{1}{5} \times 3\frac{1}{2} \times 13\frac{1}{3}$
5. $\frac{5}{14} \times 2$	*12.* $\frac{3}{4}$ of $\frac{8}{9}$	*19.* $\frac{11}{81} \times 5\frac{1}{4} \times 3\frac{3}{7}$
6. $\frac{9}{15} \times 5$	*13.* $\frac{1}{2}$ of 6	*20.* $1\frac{5}{28} \times \frac{35}{36} \times 3\frac{3}{11}$
7. $\frac{2}{5} \times 10$	*14.* $\frac{1}{3}$ of $\frac{3}{4}$	

6
Division of fractions

IT HAS been observed that a whole number can be written in fractional form by supplying it with a denominator of 1. For example, 2 in fractional form becomes $\frac{2}{1}$, 6 becomes $\frac{6}{1}$, 8 becomes $\frac{8}{1}$ and so on. This device is convenient when dealing with division in fractions.

If the fractional form of a number is turned upside down so that its denominator becomes its numerator and *vice versa*, the new fraction is called the **reciprocal** of the original fraction. For instance, 3 can be written $\frac{3}{1}$, and its reciprocal is $\frac{1}{3}$. The same is true of proper fractions. The reciprocal of $\frac{2}{7}$ is $\frac{7}{2}$; of $\frac{3}{4}$ is $\frac{4}{3}$; of $\frac{1}{2}$ is $\frac{2}{1}$.

This brings us to the rule to apply when a divisor is a fraction: **when dividing by a fraction convert the divisor into its reciprocal and multiply by it instead.** In more familiar language the rule can be stated thus: in order to divide by a fraction, turn it upside down and multiply by it. For example, in the expression $\frac{1}{3} \div \frac{2}{5}$, two fifths is the divisor. Turned upside down it becomes $\frac{5}{2}$ and the expression can be rewritten as

$$\frac{1}{3} \times \frac{5}{2}$$

It is then straightforward and equals $\frac{5}{6}$.

There is nothing more than this to the division of fractions except to state that mixed numbers must be changed to improper fractions before work starts.

Example 1: Simplify:

$$3\tfrac{1}{3} \div 7\tfrac{2}{3}$$
$$= \tfrac{10}{3} \div \tfrac{23}{3}$$
$$= \tfrac{10}{3} \times \tfrac{3}{23}$$

$$= \frac{10 \times \overset{1}{\cancel{3}}}{\cancel{3} \times 23}$$
$$\qquad \qquad 1$$
$$= \tfrac{10}{23}$$

Example 2: Divide $8\frac{1}{4}$ by $1\frac{1}{2}$

$$= 8\frac{1}{4} \div 1\frac{1}{2} = \tfrac{33}{4} \div \tfrac{3}{2} = \tfrac{33}{4} \times \tfrac{2}{3}$$
$$\quad 11 \quad \ 1$$
$$= \frac{\overset{11}{\cancel{33}} \times \overset{1}{\cancel{2}}}{\underset{2}{\cancel{4}} \times \underset{1}{\cancel{3}}} = \frac{11 \times 1}{2 \times 1} = 5\frac{1}{2}$$

Example 3: A litre and a half of milk is divided into 8 portions. What fraction of a litre is in each portion?

$$1\frac{1}{2} \div 8$$
$$= \tfrac{3}{2} \div \tfrac{8}{1}$$
$$= \tfrac{3}{2} \times \tfrac{1}{8}$$
$$= \tfrac{3}{16} \text{ of a litre in each portion.}$$

Exercises

Simplify:

1. $\frac{5}{6} \div \frac{3}{4}$	*5.* $\frac{15}{16} \div \frac{5}{4}$	*9.* $\frac{2}{3} \div \frac{3}{4}$
2. $\frac{4}{7} \div \frac{8}{9}$	*6.* $\frac{7}{8} \div 3$	*10.* $4\frac{1}{3} \div 3\frac{1}{4}$
3. $5 \div \frac{10}{11}$	*7.* $4\frac{3}{4} \div 5\frac{1}{2}$	*11.* $18 \div 1\frac{2}{7}$
4. $7 \div \frac{3}{5}$	*8.* $\frac{8}{15} \div \frac{4}{5}$	*12.* $2\frac{1}{2} \div 3\frac{1}{8}$

13. How many books each $\frac{3}{4}$ in thick can be put on a shelf 2 ft 3 in long?

14. Find the cost of 4 lb of sugar at $4\frac{1}{2}$p per lb.

15. A pint of water weighs $1\frac{1}{4}$ lb. How many pints are there in a bucket containing 35 lb of water?

16. If a nurse's stride measures $\frac{3}{5}$ metre how many steps must she take to walk from the sluice to the duty room—a distance of 18 metres?

17. By what number must $4\frac{1}{2}$ be multiplied to give a product of $1\frac{7}{8}$?

18. How many splints $\frac{3}{4}$ metre long can be cut from a board measuring $2\frac{1}{4}$ metres?

19. How many beds each $2\frac{1}{2}$ ft wide will fill a ward $42\frac{1}{2}$ ft long if there are to be two rows with a space of $5\frac{1}{2}$ ft between beds?

20. Sister is to buy rolls of crepe paper at $17\frac{1}{2}$p each. How many can she get for £2·60? How much money is left over and how many Christmas tree decorations at 5p each will this buy?

21. In order to reach a practical examination a nurse travels $\frac{4}{7}$ of the journey by car, $\frac{14}{15}$ of the rest by train and walks the last part which is $\frac{3}{4}$ mile. What is the total length of the journey?

22. A nurse sends $\frac{1}{10}$ of her month's salary home, spends $\frac{1}{30}$ of it on a new textbook, pays $\frac{1}{5}$ to her insurance agent, and banks $\frac{1}{4}$. If she then has £8·50 left, what is her monthly salary?

7

Decimal fractions

IN INFANT schools children are taught to write down numbers under certain headings—thousands, hundreds, tens and units. Later they dispense with the headings but it is worth-while recalling them and seeing what relationship they bear to each other. The number 6000 is spoken of as **six thousand**. Dividing it by ten results in a quotient of **six hundred**. Further division by ten results in sixty, which by continued use over centuries is a contraction of **six tens,** and a final division by ten results in **six units.** In the early days of a child's education this is as far as he may be taken and it is sufficient to show that each classification is ten times as great as its right-hand neighbour. Decimal notation is a means of continuing this system to include smaller numbers than units. A dot called the **decimal point** is placed after the units column and numbers are continued to the right of this point, each number representing one-tenth of the value of the numbers in the column on its immediate left. If the units 'six' are divided by ten the quotient is six-tenths, which we have seen in the chapter on fractions can be represented by $\frac{6}{10}$. It can be represented in decimals as point six which is written ·6; or more usually as 0·6 the nought being used to emphasize the decimal point and not standing for anything in particular. Without the nought the point might quite easily be overlooked.

If point six stands for $\frac{6}{10}$, division by ten would result in **six-hundredths.** The fractional form of this, $\frac{6}{100}$, is familiar but it can also be written as 0·06, the figure six now being entered in the next space after the tenths column. The process can be repeated indefinitely providing successively thousandths next to the hundredths, then ten-thousandths, then hundred-thousandths and so on.

In this way a concise method of writing down numbers without the use of denominators has been evolved. For example, the expression twenty-five, eight-tenths, seven-hundredths, three-thousandths, can be written as 25·873, and this is usually read as 'twenty-five **point** eight, seven, three'.

Exercises

Write the following fractions in decimal form:

1. $\frac{1}{10}$ *2.* $\frac{3}{10}$ *3.* $\frac{6}{10}$ *4.* $\frac{8}{100}$ *5.* $\frac{20}{100}$ *6.* $\frac{25}{100}$

From the last example it will be seen that $\frac{25}{100}$ consists of $\frac{20}{100}$ plus $\frac{5}{100}$ and by cancelling 10 in the numerator and denominator of $\frac{20}{100}$, it becomes $\frac{2}{10}$. Hence $\frac{25}{100}$ is $\frac{2}{10}$ plus $\frac{5}{100}$ and to express this as a decimal involves inserting the 2 in the tenths position and 5 in the hundredths position; 0·25.

The reverse process of converting decimals to fractions is but the work of a moment. The decimal figures are regarded as the numerator of the fraction and a denominator is supplied consisting of 1 followed by as many noughts as there are decimal figures in the numerator.

$$46·3 = 46\frac{3}{10}$$

One decimal place, therefore 1 nought in the denominator.

$$8·65 = 8\frac{65}{100}$$

Two decimal places, therefore 2 noughts in the denominator.

$$37·715 = 37\frac{715}{1000}$$

Three decimal places, therefore 3 noughts in the denominator.

For instance, the decimal 0·873 becomes $\frac{873}{1000}$; there being 3 figures in the numerator to the right of the decimal point, there must be three noughts in the denominator. (Any figures on the left of the decimal point are ignored when counting the noughts to appear in the denominator.)

Once the fraction has been discovered it may be necessary to cancel in order to present it in its lowest form.

Now regard the decimal 0·0004. It shows that there are no tenths, hundredths or thousandths, but there are four ten-thousandths which can be written as $\frac{4}{10000}$. At first glance the rule of making the decimal the numerator with as many noughts in the denominator as there are figures in the decimal seems to have broken down, but it has not in reality. The **complete** numerator should consist of all the figures to the right of the decimal point, noughts included, namely, 0004, Here there are four figures so there should be four noughts in the denominator. Once the fraction has been calculated the noughts in the numerator are dispensed with.

Example: 1. Convert each of the following to fractions reduced to their lowest terms.

(*a*) $3·1 = 3\frac{1}{10}$

(*b*) $4·6 = 4\frac{\cancel{6}^{3}}{\cancel{10}_{5}} = 4\frac{3}{5}$

(*c*) $7·45 = 7\frac{\cancel{45}^{9}}{\cancel{100}_{20}} = 7\frac{9}{20}$

(*d*) $0·05 = \frac{\cancel{5}^{1}}{\cancel{100}_{20}} = \frac{1}{20}$

(*e*) $17·875 = 17\frac{\cancel{875}^{7}}{\cancel{1000}_{8}} = 17\frac{7}{8}$

Exercises

Convert each of the following decimals into fractions in their lowest terms.

1.	5·2	*5.*	0·06		*8.*	2·55
2.	2·5	*6.*	0·006		*9.*	1·05
3.	3·25	*7.*	4·125		*10.*	0·0005
4.	0·6					

The reverse procedure of converting fractions to decimals is achieved by dividing the numerator of the fraction by its denominator. Hence to convert the fraction $\frac{1}{2}$ to a decimal, certain thoughts pass through one's head like this:

'2 into 1 won't go. Put a nought in the units column followed by a decimal point: 0·. Multiply the numerator by 10 by adding a nought to it. That makes the numerator 10. Divide this number by the denominator. 2 into 10 goes five times, with no remainder. Place the 5 next to the decimal point. Therefore $\frac{1}{2} = 0·5$.'

Example 2: Express $\frac{3}{4}$ as a decimal.

(4 into 3 won't go so put down nought followed by the decimal point.)

$$0·$$

(Multiply the numerator by 10 and divide the result by the denominator: $30 \div 4$. This goes 7 times with a remainder of 2. Place the 7 in the first decimal place.)

$$0·7$$

(Multiply the remainder by 10 and divide this by the denominator: $20 \div 4 = 5$. Place the 5 in the next decimal place.)

$$0·75$$

Therefore $\frac{3}{4} = 0·75$

Example 3: Express $\frac{3}{8}$ as a decimal.

$3 \div 8$ won't go	0·
$30 \div 8 = 3$ with 6 over	0·3

$60 \div 8 = 7$ with 4 over   0·37
$40 \div 8 = 5$ with no remainder   0·375
Therefore $\frac{3}{8} = 0·375$

Example 4: Express $\frac{7}{8}$ as a decimal.
(The working can be done most conveniently in the margin
as a simple or long division sum.)

$$\frac{7}{8} = 0·875$$

$$\begin{array}{r} 64 \\ 8)\overline{7000} \\ \overline{0875} \end{array}$$

Exercises

Express each of the following fractions in decimal form:

1. $\frac{7}{20}$	*5.* $\frac{9}{32}$	*8.* $3\frac{15}{32}$
2. $\frac{3}{25}$	*6.* $\frac{53}{80}$	*9.* $\frac{113}{40}$
3. $\frac{5}{16}$	*7.* $2\frac{13}{20}$	*10.* $\frac{432}{125}$
4. $\frac{33}{40}$		

Recurring Decimals

It is quite impossible to convert some fractions to complete
decimals. For instance, in the fraction $\frac{1}{3}$, the process of dividing
by three after multiplying each remainder by ten results in a
series of quotients of 3, and always there is another remainder
of 1. The decimal would look like this:

0·333333333333333333 ... with 1 remaining.

These are called *recurring* decimals and to indicate that
such is the case a dot is placed over the number that recurs,
thus 0·$\dot{3}$.

It occurs in many fractions particularly those with a
denominator of 3, 6, 7, 9.

An interesting type of recurrence occurs with decimals
derived from any fraction with a denominator of 7. Instead of a
single figure recurring, a whole set does so in regular order.

$\frac{1}{7} = 0·142857142857142857 \ldots$
$\frac{2}{7} = 0·2857142857142857 \ldots$
$\frac{3}{7} = 0·42857142857142857 \ldots$
$\frac{4}{7} = 0·57142857142857142857 \ldots$
$\frac{5}{7} = 0·7142857142857142857 \ldots$
$\frac{6}{7} = 0·857142857142857142857 \ldots$

It can be seen that the recurring block consists of the figures 142857. In such a case recurrence is denoted by placing a dot over both the first and last figures of the recurring block as in $\frac{4}{7} = 0.5\dot{7}14285\dot{7}$.

Such decimals can be a great nuisance in mathematics and where they occur they are best left as fractions if it is possible to do so. A fraction is always complete and exact whereas a recurring decimal is an approximation. Fortunately recurring decimals rarely occur in nursing problems.

Significant Figures

Sometimes information need only be expressed to the nearest 100 or nearest 1000, etc. For example, if the population of an area was said to be 282,912 the sum might be rounded off and expressed as 283,000 to three significant figures or as 282,900 to four significant figures.

Decimal places can be similarly treated. Thus, 0·2428 expressed to three decimal places would be 0·243. Again, 2·756 would be 2·76 if expressed to three significant figures or 2·8 if expressed to two significant figures.

Noughts in a whole number are not counted as significant figures unless they are between non-zero digits; neither are the noughts between the decimal point and the first non-zero digit counted as significant decimal places.

Multiplication in Decimals

(1) Copy the expression carefully on to the paper.
(2) Work out a rough answer using approximate values of the numbers instead of decimals.
(3) Ignore the decimal points and multiply the numbers as if they were ordinary whole numbers.
(4) Write down the product as a whole number.
(5) Add up the total number of decimal places in the numbers as written in rule (1).

(6) Starting at the right-hand figure in the product as written under rule (4), count as many figures as there are decimal places under rule (5).
(7) Place the decimal point in front of that many figures.
(8) Check with the rough answer made in rule (2) to see if the answer is feasible.

These rules will be clearer if a few examples are worked.

Example 1: Simply 0·5 × 3·2

Rule (1)   0·5 × 3·2
Rule (2)   (rough answer 0·5 × 3 = 1·5)
Rule (3)   5 × 32
Rule (4)   = 160
Rule (5)   There is a total of two decimal places, one from the 0·5 and one from the 3·2
Rule (6) and Rule (7)   Starting with the right-hand figure, count two places and insert the decimal point to the left of the second, 1·60.
Rule (8)   Check with the rough answer to make sure that the answer is feasible. (In this case the final nought can be omitted once the position of the decimal point has been established, but not before.)

Example 2: Simplify 7·46 × 3·2 × 14·7

Rough answer 7 × 3 × 15 = 315

746 × 32 × 147   (This may be worked by long multiplication in the margin.)

= 3509184   (Decimal places total 4, two from 7·46 one from 3·2, and one from 14·7. Therefore the decimal point is placed in front of the fourth figure from the right.)

350·9184   (Which agrees with the rough answer.)

$$\begin{array}{r} 746 \\ 32 \\ \hline 1492 \\ 2238 \\ \hline 23872 \\ 147 \\ \hline 167104 \\ 95488 \\ 23872 \\ \hline 3509184 \end{array}$$

Example 3: Multiply together 2·9, 0·58, 1·03

Rough answer 3 × 0·5 × 1 = 1·5

29 × 58 × 103

= 173246   (5 decimal places)

1·73246

$$\begin{array}{r} 29 \\ 58 \\ \hline 232 \\ 145 \\ \hline 1682 \\ 103 \\ \hline 5046 \\ 1682 \\ \hline 173246 \end{array}$$

Sometimes the product of two or more decimals does not contain enough figures to apply the rule for the correct placing of the decimal point. In such a case enough figures are created by placing noughts to the left of the figures in the product. For instance 0·5 × 0·005 gives a product of 25 and the decimal point must be placed in front of the fourth figure. Obviously there are only two figures in 25, but by placing two noughts in front of them there will be no alteration in their value but it will then be possible to place the decimal point in its correct place: ·0025.

Multiplying decimals by 10 is perhaps the easiest task possible to perform as it merely involves shifting the decimal place one position to the right. For instance, 5 × 10 as everyone knows is 50. If we express 5 as 5·0 it will be seen that in the product, the decimal point has moved one place to the right. Similarly, right throughout decimals this is possible:

$$0·005 × 10 = 0·05$$

When multiplying by 100 the decimal point is moved **two** places to the right. This is quite clear if 100 is looked upon as consisting of 10 × 10. Multiplying by 10 involves moving the decimal one place to the right, therefore multiplying by two tens involves moving the decimal two places to the right.

Multiplying by 1000 involves three shifts to the right as 1000 equals 10 × 10 × 10, and so on.

In this fact lies the beauty of the metric system in which all measurements are in units that have one-tenth of the value of the next highest measure. 1 decimetre is $\frac{1}{10}$ of a metre, 1 milligram is $\frac{1}{10}$ of a centigram, etc.

Exercises

1.   Multiply each of the following by 10.

(a)   0·7   (b)   1·7   (c)   0·007   (d)   3·04   (e)   7·32

2.   Multiply each of the following by 100.

(a)   3·2   (b)   17·04   (c)   0·007   (d)   1·007   (e)   13·1

3. 4·83 × 0·3	*10.* 8·3 × 0·011
4. 37·4 × 0·5	*11.* 0·077 × 0·03
5. 2413 × 0·04	*12.* 3·24 × 8·46
6. 0·73 × 0·8	*13.* 37·4 × 0·05483
7. 3·142 × 0·7	*14.* 7·5 × 0·75 × 0·075
8. 0·83 × 1·1	*15.* 92 × 0·31 × 2·3
9. 0·83 × 0·11	*16.* 36·9 × 1·014 × 2·5

Division in Decimals

Consider the following expression: Three divided by four. This can be written in fractional form $\frac{3}{4}$ as has been seen in the chapter on fractions. Similarly, the expression:

point five divided by point two five

can be written in fractional form

$$\frac{0·5}{0·25}$$

It will be remembered that fractions can be expanded by multiplying both the numerator and the denominator by equal amounts. The resulting fraction may not look anything like the original, but it has exactly the same value. This principle can be used to great advantage when dealing with expressions such as that written above.

$$\frac{0·5}{0·25} \text{ looks ugly}$$

If the numerator and the denominator is multiplied by 100 it becomes $\frac{50}{25}$. It looks nothing like the original but we know it has the same value and is a much more manageable expression. Clearly 50 divided by 25 equals 2.

It is only necessary to convert the denominator into a whole number. The denominator is the number that is going to be used to do the dividing and is called a **divisor**. If this is in whole number form the division can progress in the margin in simple or long form whichever is more convenient, even if the numerator still has a decimal point in it. Hence, the expression:

divide 1·326 by 0·3

rewritten in fractional form becomes

$$\frac{1·326}{0·3}$$

Multiplying top and bottom by 10 makes it

$$\frac{13·26}{3}$$

$$\frac{3 \overline{)13·26}}{4·42}$$

a simple division sum.

A rule for the division of decimals can now be formulated.

To divide by a decimal, rewrite the expression as a fraction and multiply the numerator and the denominator by a number sufficient to convert the denominator into a whole number.

It is wise not to omit rewriting the expression as a fraction until the multiplication is fully grasped, but that step can be left out once confidence has been gained.

Example 1: Divide 17·943 by 0·25

$$= \frac{17·943}{0·25} \quad \text{(multiply top and bottom by 100)}$$

$$= \frac{1794·3}{25}$$

$$= 71·772$$

$$\frac{5 \overline{)1794·3}}{5 \overline{)358·86}}$$
$$\overline{71·772}$$

Example 2: Simplify 0·072 ÷ 0·0012

$$= \frac{0·072}{0·0012} \quad \text{(multiply top and bottom by 10,000)}$$

$$= \frac{720}{12}$$

$$= 60$$

Example 3: Divide 27·42 by 0·032

$$= \frac{27·42}{0·032} \quad \text{(multiply top and bottom by 1,000)}$$

$$= \frac{27420}{32}$$

$$= 856·875$$

8)27420
4)3427·5
856·875

Exercises

1. Express the following as decimals of 1 litre:

  (*a*) 50 millilitres (*b*) 2 decilitres (*c*) 30 centilitres

2. Express the following as decimals of £2

        (*a*) 10p (*b*) 25p (*c*) 37½p (*d*) 30p

3. Express the following as decimals of 1 litre:

(*a*) 100 ml   (*b*) 40 ml   (*c*) 840 ml   (*d*) 1 ml

4. Express as decimals or whole numbers:

(*a*)	0·45 ÷ 0·5	(*f*)	5·0008 ÷ 89·3
(*b*)	0·44 ÷ 1·1	(*g*)	0·76107 ÷ 0·23
(*c*)	0·32 ÷ 0·08	(*h*)	0·0032 ÷ 0·08
(*d*)	0·0066 ÷ 0·6	(*i*)	12·63 ÷ 0·3
(*e*)	12 ÷ 0·04	(*j*)	25 ÷ 0·5

5. Multiply each of the following by 10, 100, 1000:

(*a*) 9·9   (*b*) 8·79   (*c*) 0·6   (*d*) 0·01   (*e*) 0·65
(*f*) 0·408 (*g*) 93·28 (*h*) 7·05 (*i*) 40·02

6. Divide each of the following by 10, 100, 1000:

(*a*) 750   (*b*) 62·32   (*c*) 4·23   (*d*) 0·025

7. Write down as decimals:

      (*a*) $\frac{72}{10}$ (*b*) $\frac{93}{100}$ (*c*) $\frac{12}{1000}$ (*d*) $\frac{7008}{100}$

8. Express the following decimals in fractional form in their lowest terms (or as mixed numbers where appropriate):

(a) 0·9   (b) 0·09   (c) 0·25 (d) 2·25   (e) 0·448
(f) 2·076 (g) 0·0025

9.   Simplify each of the following expressions:

(a) 2·5 × 0·023   (b) 0·006 × 1·08   (c) 32·75 × 4·8
(d) 11·81 × 4·2   (e) 39·44 × 2·3   (f) 4·29 × 61·12

10.   Express as recurring decimals:

(a) $\frac{1}{3}$ (b) $\frac{5}{6}$ (c) $\frac{1}{9}$ (d) $\frac{3}{11}$ (e) $\frac{1}{7}$

11.   Express the following to three significant figures:

(a) 24,780 (b) 275,999   (c) 975,900

express the following to two significant decimal places:

(d) 0·00758 (e) 0·8768   (f) 0·0939   (g) 0·06717

Problems

12.   If 4·5 litres of milk is supplied to a 20-bed ward how much is allowed per patient? Express the answer in (a) litres, (b) decilitres, (c) millilitres.

13.   6·45 tons of coal are consumed by a boiler in 30 days. How much is needed for 1 week?

14.   How many trays with an area of 2·25 square feet can be laid on a table with an area of 52·75 square feet?

15.   If a bank pays £2·50 sterling interest on each £100 deposited for 1 year, how much interest will a nurse get who leaves £270·32 in the bank for 3 years? (Simple interest).

16.   The analysis written on a patent food packet states

0·7   parts carbohydrate
0·25 parts protein
0·05 parts fat

What weight of each is present in a 500-gramme packet?

17.   If 0·75 parts of the staff of a hospital are to be on duty at all times, how many nurses can be off at once with a staff of 40?

8
Decimal currency

£.s.d. CURRENCY has had a long and turbulent history. The letter 'd' was the symbol for a denarius, an old Roman coin that was sometimes called a penny, hence its use as a symbol for English pennies. Dating from the eighth century, one pound weight (troy) of silver was divided into 240 parts, each called a penny. For a long time the silver penny was the only commonly used coin. Later on, copper was used for coins of small denomination, but these became uneconomical, were discredited by clipping and were eventually withdrawn from circulation. Bronze pennies were introduced in 1860. Pounds and shillings were not minted until the reign of Henry VII, the shilling being one-twentieth of a pound.

French currency was decimalized when the metric system was introduced, and in 1792 the U.S.A. adopted a decimal system based on the dollar. Most European countries adopted decimal systems during the Nineteenth Century and since then many Commonwealth countries have followed suit. The introduction of the florin in 1849 was the first step taken in England towards a decimal system; until 1887 florins were inscribed as 'one-tenth of a pound'. Eventually the Government decided to decimalize the English currency and the Royal Mint was authorized to mint a new coinage, which became legal currency on 15th February 1971.

The pound sterling has been retained as the fundamental unit of our currency. £1 is now divided into 100 equal parts, each part being known for the time being as a 'new penny' with the symbol 'p' used to differentiate it from the old penny. The new halfpenny is the smallest unit of decimal currency; it is denoted by the vulgar fraction $\frac{1}{2}$p. £1 is the smallest denomination for which a currency note can be obtained; sums less than £1 can only be paid in coins. Apart from the ½p and 1p there are 2p, 5p, 10p and 50p coins.

When writing down sums greater than £1 the correct method is to write each sum as a whole number and a decimal of a pound. Thus, £12·75 is correct whereas £12·75p is wrong; the latter sum could be interpreted as being 12·75 pence. Sums less than one pound can be written either as a decimal of a pound or as a number of pence. Thus, 25 pence can be written as £0·25 or as 25p. Normally halfpennies should be written as vulgar fractions after the decimal sum, e.g. 75½p; £1·24½p. For the purpose of making calculations halfpennies can be written as a third decimal and then expressed as a vulgar fraction in the answer.

Example:

$$£1·34\tfrac{1}{2} \times 7 = £1·345$$
$$\underline{7}$$
$$\overline{9·415} = £9·41\tfrac{1}{2}$$

When writing a cheque a hyphen is used instead of a decimal point in order to reduce the risk of error. As banks will not pay out halfpennies on cheques the sum has to be rounded off to the nearest whole penny. Two figures should always be placed after the hyphen, otherwise an amount such as £2-6. could be taken as being either 2 pounds and 60 pence, or as 2 pounds and 6 pence (£2-06). When whole pounds are being paid the amount in figures should be followed by a hyphen and two noughts or by a long dash; the sum in words should be followed by the word 'only'.

Examples:

Amount in words	*Amount in figures*
Five pounds 26	£5-26
Seven pounds 06	£7-06
Eight pounds only———	£8-00 or £8———
Twenty-five pence	£0-25 or 25p

When calculations in decimal currency have been made we may be left with a fraction of 1p that could be greater or less than one-halfpenny. In such cases the final result should be corrected to obtain an answer to the nearest $\frac{1}{2}$p. Calculations should be taken to the fourth place only if it is doubtful whether the corrected answer should be $\frac{1}{2}$p more or $\frac{1}{2}$p less. Usually when engaged in simple sums of addition or subtraction the halfpennies can be expressed as vulgar fractions.

Example 1: Add £1·77$\frac{1}{2}$; £12; 48p; 71$\frac{1}{2}$p; £3·40$\frac{1}{2}$

$$1·77\tfrac{1}{2}$$
$$12·00$$
$$0·48$$
$$0·71\tfrac{1}{2}$$
$$3·40\tfrac{1}{2}$$

Answer: £18·37$\frac{1}{2}$

Example 2: Subtract £19·07$\frac{1}{2}$ from £26·15

$$26·15$$
$$19·07\tfrac{1}{2}$$

Answer: £7·07$\frac{1}{2}$

Example 3: Evaluate

$$£12·85\tfrac{1}{2} \times 52·7$$
$$12·855$$
$$52·7$$
$$642·75$$
$$25·710$$
$$8·9985$$
$$£677·4585$$

The answer corrected to the nearest $\frac{1}{2}$p is **£677·46**

Example 4: Fifteen milligrams of a carcino-chemotherapeutic drug costs £58·62. What is the cost of 1 mg to the nearest 1p?

$$\begin{array}{r} 3 \cdot 908 \\ 15\overline{)58 \cdot 62} \\ \underline{45} \\ 136 \\ \underline{135} \\ 120 \\ \underline{120} \end{array}$$

The cost of 1 mg to the nearest 1p is **£3·91.**

When dividing a number by another decimal number difficulty is reduced by multiplying both numbers by ten, or multiples of ten, so that the divisor is a whole number.

Example: £55·35 earned from a work project is to be divided among 12 people who have each worked 10 hours and another person who has worked for only 3 hours. What should each receive?

12 people worked for the whole time and another for 0·3 of the time, therefore the amount paid for 10 hours work is £55·35 ÷ 12·3. Multiplying both numbers by ten produces £553·5 ÷ 123.

$$\begin{array}{r} 4 \cdot 5 \\ 123\overline{)553 \cdot 5} \\ \underline{492} \\ 615 \\ \underline{615} \end{array}$$

Thus, those who worked 10 hours each earned £4·50
The earnings for 3 hours work amount to:

$$\frac{4 \cdot 50 \times 3}{10} = \textbf{£1·35}$$

Exercises

Add the following:

1. £3·95; £7·05; £133·50; 50p
2. £17·09; £20·81; £7·10; £291·85½
3. £35·30; £67·05; £73·16; £38·12

Evaluate:

4. £133·09 − £26·59½
5. £189·40 − £132·72

Multiply:

6. £98·03½ by 12
7. £67·07½ by 7·4

Divide:

8. £4·09½ by 9
9. £160·50 by 15
10. What is ⅔ of £269·10?
11. What is 12½% of £1160·00?
12. Each week a ward is supplied with 12 daily papers at 3p a copy; 8 Sunday papers at 4p each; 6 magazines at 15p each and 7 magazines at 20p each. What is the total expenditure in a 4-week period?

Foreign Exchange

Converting foreign money into English money is much less complex when both currencies are based upon a decimal system. However, the tourist is faced with greater uncertainty now that the U.S.A. dollar has been taken off the Gold Standard and more foreign currencies are being allowed to float. Travellers can no longer always be certain that a given sum can be converted into a predetermined number of units of foreign currency. The rate of exchange, which is simply the price of foreign money, can go up or down according to the rates of supply and demand unless there is an exchange control.

The following table is an example of some of the exchange rates in January 1972. Nurses going abroad should consult the financial sections of their newspapers to see how much foreign money their savings will buy.

Country	Currency units	Rate of exchange for £1
France	1 Franc = 100 centimes	13·29 francs
Belgium	1 Franc = 100 cents	114·00 francs
West Germany	1 Deutsche Mark = 100 pfennige	8·31 D.M.
Switzerland	1 Franc = 100 centimes	10·00 francs
Italy	1 Lira = 100 centisimi	1520·00 lire
Spain	1 Peseta = 100 centimos	170·5 pesetas
Canada	1 Dollar ($) = 100 cents	2·6 dollars
U.S.A.	1 Dollar ($) = 100 cents	2·58 dollars

When money is exchanged sums are rounded off to the nearest whole unit, when bank charges are deducted. Bank charges have been ignored in the following examples.

Example 1: A woman has saved £70 for a holiday. How much will she obtain in: (*a*) French, (*b*) Belgian, and (*c*) Canadian currencies? Use the exchange rates in the table above.

(*a*)   £1 = 13·29 francs. $70 \times 13 \cdot 29 = 930 \cdot 3$
            therefore £70 = 930·3 francs (French)

(*b*)   £1 = 114·00 francs. $70 \times 114 \cdot 00 = 7980 \cdot 00$
        therefore £70 = 7980·00 francs (Belgian)

(*c*)   £1 = $2·6
            therefore £70 = 2·6 dollars (Canadian) × 70
                = 182 dollars (Canadian)

Example 2: A man goes on a study tour in North America. He takes £400 with him and converts this into dollars at an exchange rate of $2·45⅞. His expenses amounted to 533 dollars and 50 cents. How much English money can he obtain on his return if the exchange rate is now $2·45¼?

$$£1 = \$2 \cdot 45\tfrac{7}{8} \quad (0 \cdot 00\tfrac{7}{8} = 0 \cdot 00875)$$

therefore £400 = 2·45875

$$\begin{array}{r} \times \quad 400 \\ \hline 983 \cdot 50000 \end{array} = 983 \text{ dollars, 50 cents.}$$

His expenses amounted to $533·50 therefore the balance amounts to:

$$\begin{array}{r} 983 \cdot 50 \\ -533 \cdot 50 \\ \hline 450 \cdot 00 \text{ dollars} \end{array}$$

On return to England the exchange rate is $2·45¼

$$\$ = \frac{£1}{2 \cdot 45\tfrac{1}{4}} = \frac{1}{2 \cdot 4525}$$

the decimal point can be removed by multiplying by 400.

$$\left[\frac{1}{2 \cdot 4525} \times \frac{4}{4} = \frac{4}{9 \cdot 81} \times \frac{100}{100} = \frac{400}{981} \right]$$

therefore $450 = $\dfrac{400 \times 450}{981}$ £ = $\dfrac{180,000}{981}$ = £183·486

thus $450 will buy **£183·48½**

Exercises

1. An English tourist in Italy paid 9450 lire for a gift to bring home. What is the cost in pounds if £1 = 1512 lire?

2. A motorist plans a journey in France of 200 kilometres a day for 5 days. The cost of travel is calculated to be 0·27½ francs for each kilometre, plus 82·50 francs a day for other expenses. How many pounds sterling will he need to convert to francs for his journey if the rate of exchange is 13·75 francs to £1?

3. If 1 guilder is worth 180 lire and 1520 lire is equal to £1, how many guilders can be bought for £45?

4. Fifty tablets of a drug in West Germany cost D.M. 0·42.

How much would a hospital in the United Kingdom have to pay to import 10,000 tablets? (D.M. 8·40 = £1).

5. Six kilogrammes of fruit in Spain cost 336·60 pesetas. How much is this in English money per lb (weight) if the exchange rate is 170 pesetas to £1? (1 kg = 2·2 lb).

6. Total purchases in America amount to the equivalent of 248 dollars. Import duty is 20% on half the articles (124 dollars) and 30% on the other half. What is the total cost in pounds sterling? (£1 = $2·50).

9
The metric system

OPINION in favour of adopting the metric system in preference to the older English systems of measurement has been gaining strength for many years. It has been argued that there are many advantages to be obtained by using the same methods of measurement that are used by most other countries. This is particularly important as closer economic, social and political links are established between the United Kingdom and Western Europe.

There is also much to commend the discarding of lengthy and poorly understood methods for simpler ones, providing there is no loss of efficiency. Such views were held by the rulers of France at the end of the eighteenth century for it was they who introduced the metric system into Europe in a successful bid to simplify matters. In that era there was not merely a few units of measurement to confuse the populace, there were no fewer than 200 standards of weight alone and no matter how conservative one's views may be it is obvious that such a state of affairs could not have been allowed to continue.

In 1790 an invitation was extended from France to this country to share in a common metric system of weights and measures, but no action was taken. However, in Europe and elsewhere the metric system gained rapid acceptance. An international treaty, the Metre Convention, was signed by seventeen countries in 1875, and by the United Kingdom in 1884. More than 90% of the world's people are now using the metric system of measurement.

Following a request from the Federation of British Industries in 1965 the Government finally agreed to introduce the metric system; 1975 was set as the target date for completion of the changeover. To assist in the changeover the Metrication Board was set up in 1969.

Official adoption of the metric system by the National Health Service for handling pharmaceutical preparations was an important step in the process of metrication. Once nurses became accustomed to administering medicines in metric doses they quickly realized that the metric system is easier to understand than traditional English weights and measures.

There is one basic unit for each property to be measured such as weight or volume. The size of a unit can be expressed in terms of multiples of tens or tenths of other units. Thus, expression of measurements in terms of higher or lower units becomes easy as only an adjustment of the decimal point is required. Further, the units are based on some definite, measurable and fixed standard and not, as previously, on some variable and ill-defined quantity like the length of an arm from elbow to finger tip, or the weight of a grain of wheat.

The distance unit is the metre. This is the length of a bar of platinum–iridium at a temperature of 0°C, kept at the International Bureau of Weights and Measures in France.

The unit of weight is the gramme, which was defined as the weight of one cubic centimetre of water at 4°C at sea level. The unit is now based on the mass of a cylinder of platinum–iridium.

The unit of volume is the litre, which is the volume occupied by one kilogram of water, once again at 4°C. It is approximately equal to 1000 cubic centimetres. (The exact volume of a kilogram of water at maximum density is 1·000028 cubic decimetre.)

Multiples of the basic measurements occur in steps of ten. The same principle applies to fractions of the base unit. A prefix indicates the enhanced or diminished value of the basic unit.

Prefix	Factor	Symbol
mega	one million times	M
kilo	one thousand times	k
hecto*	one hundred times	h
deca *	ten times	da
deci *	one-tenth	d
centi *	one-hundredth	c
milli	one-thousandth	m
micro	one-millionth	μ

The prefixes marked * are normally not used in everyday matters. The accepted symbols are shown above, but it is always wise to write terms in full whenever an error could lead to serious consequences. Consideration of the symbols M and m; k and h; da and d; clearly reveal the danger of not writing symbols legibly, if they are to be used at all.

Using these prefixes, tables are built up as follows:

Distance

10 millimetres (mm)	= 1 centimetre	(cm)
10 centimetres	= 1 decimetre	(dm)
10 decimetres	= 1 *metre*	(m)
10 metres	= 1 decametre	(dam)
10 decametres	= 1 hectometre	(hm)
10 hectometres	= 1 kilometre	(km)

Weight

10 milligram (mg)	= 1 centigram	(cg)
10 centigrams	= 1 decigram	(dg)
10 decigrams	= 1 *gramme*	(g)
10 grammes	= 1 decagram	(dag)
10 decagrams	= 1 hectogram	(hg)
10 hectograms	= 1 kilogram	(kg)
1000 kilograms	= 1 tonne	(t)

The accepted symbol for a gramme in prescription writing is G. In all other cases the international symbol g should be used. The word gramme is frequently shortened to gram when accompanied by a prefix in prescriptions.

Area

    100 square millimetres = 1 square centimetre   (cm²)
    100 square centimetres = 1 square decimetre   (dm²)
    100 square decimetres = 1 *square metre*   (m²)
    100 square metres   = 1 square decametre   (dam²)
    100 square decametres = 1 square hectometre   (hm²)
    100 square hectometres = 1 square kilometre   (km²)

The ARE is the unit for measuring the area of land. Thus:
1 hectare (ha) = 100 ares   = 1 square hectometre.
1 are (a)   = 1 square decametre = 100 square metres.

Volume

1000 cubic millimetres (mm³) = 1 cubic centimetre (cm³)
1000 cubic centimetres   = 1 cubic decimetre   (dm³)
1000 cubic decimetres   = 1 cubic metre   (m³)

Different terms are used to describe measurements of capacity, although these are linked to volume as shown below.

Capacity

10 millilitres (ml) = 1 centilitre   (cl)
10 centilitres   = 1 decilitre   (dl)
10 decilitres   = 1 *litre*   (l) = 1 cubic decimetre
                                             (dm³) (approxi-
                                             mately)
10 litres   = 1 decalitre   (dal)
10 decalitres   = 1 hectolitre   (hl)

The international symbols have been shown and the danger of confusing these with one another will again have been noticed. It cannot be stressed too strongly that terms should be written in full whenever the consequences of error would be serious.

Measuring the Very Small

Many substances used in medicine in these modern times have to be measured in exceedingly small doses. To eliminate the use of fractions and decimals the prefixes micro; nano; pico; femto; and atto have been introduced. The first of these prefixes is the only one likely to be needed by nurses. For example, a microgram is one-thousandth of a milligram (0·000001 g). It can be abbreviated to μg (the greek letter mu), but this looks so similar to mg for milligram that it is better to write it in full.

Similarly microscopic distances are better expressed in whole numbers rather than decimal points followed by strings of noughts. Thus a micron is one-thousandth of a millimetre, which, if you have a ruler graduated in centimetres and millimetres before you, you will agree is an exceedingly small distance. One of the smallest micro-organisms visible through an ordinary microscope is the virus of smallpox. This is about 0·2 microns (micrometres, μm) in diameter. Red blood cells are about 7 microns in diameter and about 2 microns in thickness. See how much easier it is to say and write this than to say that red blood cells are 0·007 mm in diameter and 0·002 mm in thickness.

Exercises

Complete the following sums:

1. 1 g = ...mg
2. 1 litre = ...ml
3. 3155 mm = ...m
4. 250 ml = ... litre
5. 1500 mg = ...g
6. 1·75 litre = ... ml
7. 48·56 ml = ...litre
8. 1·08 litre = ...ml
9. 15 ml = ...cm³
10. 100 cm³ = ... ml
11. 0·062 g = ...mg
12. 960 ml = ...litre
13. 45·9 ml = ...litre
14. 9·6 kg = ...g
15. 40 litres + 364 ml = ...litre
16. 32 mg + 760 mg + 480 mg = ...g

17. 8 litres − 469 ml = ...litre........ml
18. 0·54 mg + 920 mg + 663·mg − 1·56 g =
     ....mg = ...g
19. 0·75 mg = ...μg
20. 750 microns = ... mm

Conversion from One Scale to Another

Some departments in a hospital, such as the laboratory and
the pharmacy, are now using metric measurements almost
exclusively. However, use is still being made of imperial
measures for many items that are used in the wards. Until
metric measures are used for all everyday affairs it will be
necessary for the nurse to be able to convert from one system
to another.

Usually it is impossible to state **exactly** what a unit in one
scale is in terms of the units of another. The best that can
be achieved is an approximation. For instance, one can state
that a metre equals 39·4 inches. For most everyday purposes
this would be quite adequate, but if one wanted greater
accuracy one could use the figure of 39·37, or closer still—
39·369, or even 39·3693. In other words it is possible to go on
adding decimal places making the approximation closer and
closer but never arriving at a figure which is the exact equivalent of 1 metre. It is the same with all other such conversion
figures.

The important question in all conversions from one scale
into another is, 'How accurate must I be?' If a nurse were
asked to measure a patient's leg for the fitting of a caliper
and to give the measurement in metric units, she might, if
she were unwise, measure with an inch tape measure and then
convert to metres by using the conversion figure of 39·3693.
This would give an answer that would be very exact but would
be more exact than the makers of the caliper could work to.
As the accuracy of the apparatus is rarely closer than the
nearest tenth of an inch the nurse need merely have used the

conversion figure of 39·4, thus saving herself a considerable amount of mental effort and reducing the risk of error considerably.

In all the following paragraphs a working conversion figure is given. This should be adequate for almost all conversions met with in the ordinary course of events in the wards. Given in brackets is a more accurate figure which can be used if a very close approximation is required.

Now that pharmaceutical preparations are not prescribed in grains and minims the nurse is most unlikely to need to convert these measures into milligrams and millilitres. A table of equivalent metric and imperial doses is given in the Appendix (p. 196), should these be required.

Measures of length

Inches and centimetres

1 inch (in) = $2\frac{1}{2}$ centimetres (cm) (2·54 cm)

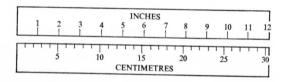

To convert inches to centimetres multiply by $\frac{5}{2}$.
To convert centimetres to inches multiply by $\frac{2}{5}$.

The degree of accuracy achieved with this figure is within one-fifth of an inch for every foot. For example:

12 inches = $12 \times \frac{5}{2}$ = 30 centimetres using the $2\frac{1}{2}$ conversion figure.

12 inches = $12 \times 2\cdot54$ = 30·48 centimetres using the 2·54 conversion figure.

Hence there is undervaluation of nearly $\frac{1}{2}$ a centimetre which is almost exactly one-fifth of an inch. It would be wise, therefore, to add one-fifth of an inch to every foot when converting to centimetres and to subtract that amount for every 30 centimetres when converting to inches.

Millimetres and Inches

1 millimetre = $\frac{1}{25}$ inch (0·039 in)

> *To convert millimetres to inches multiply by $\frac{1}{25}$.*
> *To convert inches to millimetres muliply by 25.*

Measurement of blood pressure is expressed in millimetres of mercury. This is explained fully in Chapter 16 (p. 145).

To get a clear picture of the length of a millimetre take an ordinary ruler that is graduated in metric units along one edge. Usually there is a blank stretch about 4 inches long. This is a decimetre, which is one-tenth part of a metre. Decimetres are not used very much. Next there is another decimetre divided into ten sections, each of which is a centimetre. Next, each centimetre is divided into ten equal sections and each one is a millimetre.

Example 1: How many millimetres must be cut from a sheet of paper 21 centimetres long to make it fit into a book 6 inches long?

$$6 \text{ inches} = 6 \times 25 \text{ mm} = 150 \text{ mm}$$
$$21 \text{ cm} = 210 \text{ mm}$$
$$\therefore \text{ Length to be removed} = 210 - 150 \text{ mm}$$
$$= 60 \text{ mm}$$

Example 2: A patient's blood pressure has been expressed as '5 inches systolic'.

Express this in the more usual form, in millimetres

$$5 \text{ inches} = 5 \times 25 \text{ mm} = 125 \text{ mm}$$
$$\therefore \text{ the blood pressure} = 125 \text{ mm systolic}$$

Measures of Weight

Kilograms and Pounds

1 kilogram (kg) = $2\frac{1}{5}$ pounds (lb) (2·205 lb)

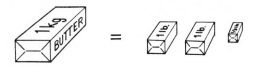

1 kilogram = $2\frac{1}{5}$ pounds

To convert kilograms to pounds multiply by $\frac{11}{5}$.
To convert pounds to kilograms multiply by $\frac{5}{11}$.

Example 1: If a patient weighs 65 kg what is this in stones and pounds?

$$65 \text{ kg} = 65 \times \tfrac{11}{5} \text{ lb}$$
$$= 13 \times 11 \text{ lb}$$
$$= 143 \text{ lb}$$
$$= 10 \text{ st } 3 \text{ lb}$$

Example 2: What is 1 cwt in kilograms?

$$1 \text{ cwt} = 112 \text{ lb} = 112 \times \tfrac{5}{11} \text{ kg}$$
$$= \tfrac{560}{11} \text{ kg}$$
$$= 51 \text{ kg approximately.}$$

(The round figures 1 cwt = 50 kg are often used for quick calculation.)

Measures of Volume

Fluid Drachms and Millilitres

1 fluid drachm (fl dr) = $3\frac{1}{2}$ millilitres (3·5515 ml)

To convert fluid drachms to millilitres multiply by $\frac{7}{2}$.
To convert millilitres to fluid drachms multiply by $\frac{2}{7}$.

Example 1: If the daily dose of cod liver oil is 2 fl dr, how much should be measured out if a millilitre measure only is available?

$$2 \text{ fl dr} = 2 \times \tfrac{7}{2} \text{ ml}$$
$$= 7 \text{ ml}$$

Therefore 7 ml should be measured out.

Example 2: How many fluid drachms of nikethamide are contained in an ampoule labelled 4 ml?

$$4 \text{ ml} = 4 \times \tfrac{2}{7} \text{ fl dr}$$
$$= 1\tfrac{1}{7} \text{ fl dr}$$

Therefore there is $1\tfrac{1}{7}$ fl dr.

Litres and Fluid Ounces

1 litre (l) = 35 fluid ounces (fl oz) (35·196 fl oz)

To convert litres to fluid ounces multiply by 35.
To convert fluid ounces to litres multiply by $\tfrac{1}{35}$.

Example 1: A pint of water weighs $1\tfrac{1}{4}$ lb. What does a litre weigh in ounces (Avoirdupois)?

$$1 \text{ pint} = 20 \text{ fl oz} = \overset{4}{\cancel{20}} \times \frac{1}{\underset{7}{\cancel{35}}} \text{ litres}$$

$$= \tfrac{4}{7} \text{ l}$$

Therefore $\tfrac{4}{7}$ of a litre weighs $1\tfrac{1}{4}$ lb.
Therefore 1 litre weighs $1\tfrac{1}{4} \times \tfrac{7}{4}$ lb.

$$= \frac{5}{\underset{1}{\cancel{4}}} \times \frac{7}{\underset{1}{\cancel{4}}} \times \overset{\overset{1}{}\overset{4}{}}{\cancel{16}} \text{ oz} \quad (1 \text{ lb} = 16 \text{ oz})$$

$$= 35 \text{ oz}$$

Example 2: If an arm bath is to contain 5 litres of saline and you have only a pint measure, how much will you measure out?

$$5 \text{ litres} = 5 \times 35 \text{ fl oz}$$

$$= \frac{\overset{1}{\cancel{5}} \times 35}{\underset{4}{\cancel{20}}} \text{ pints}$$

$$= \tfrac{35}{4} \text{ pints}$$

$$= 8\tfrac{3}{4} \text{ pints}$$

Therefore you would measure out $8\tfrac{3}{4}$ pints.

Exercises

1. Convert each of the following to (i) kilograms, (ii) pounds.

(a) 0·5 g × 450   (b) 177·5 g × 20

(c) 6·5 g × 34   (d) 400 × 3·5

2. Express each of the following in (i) kilograms, (ii) grammes.

(a) $\tfrac{1}{2}$ lb   (b) 10 lb   (c) 2·2 lb

(d) $5\tfrac{1}{2}$ lb

(work to 3 decimal places only).

3. Kilograms and pounds.

In a class, six of the pupils weigh 40, 48, 56, 58, 62 and 100 kg.

(a) Express each of these weights in stones and pounds.

(b) What is the average weight of these six in kilograms and in pounds?

4. Calculate the total quantity of the following drugs consumed by an average of ten people, for each drug, in: (a) millilitres and (b) litres. Doses given are for one person.

(i) Largactil syrup 10 ml, three times a day for 4 weeks.

(ii) Potassium citrate (BNF) 10 ml, three times a day for 5 days.

(*iii*) Aluminium hydroxide mixture 5 ml three times a day for 3 weeks.

(*iv*) Chloral hydrate (BNF) 20 ml once a day for 2 weeks.

5. Fluid drachms and millilitres.

(*a*) Convert each of the following to millilitres:

  8 20 34 $\frac{1}{4}$ 3 fl dr

(*b*) Convert each of the following to fluid drachms:

  7·2 9 56 49 100 ml

6. Litres and fluid ounces.

(*a*) Express the following in pints and fluid ounces:

40 ml 100 ml 1·5 litres 500 ml 375 ml

(*b*) Express the following in litres or millilitres:

  1 pint 2 fl oz 3 fl dr $\frac{1}{2}$ fl oz

7. The daily dosage of streptomycin is expressed as 20 milligrams per kilogram of body weight.

What would the dosage be for a man weighing 60 kilograms?

8. Arrange the following in size order of weight:

  1086 mg, 0·75 kg, 1 lb, 0·8 g

9. Arrange the following in size order of volume:

  0·5 litre, 0·75 pint, 180 fl oz, 625 ml, 300 cc

Conversion Tables

Tables 1 to 3 are ready reckoners which make conversion much easier. They contain, however, approximate conversions only and therefore the answers obtained from them are not very accurate, particularly when comparatively large numbers are being converted. To use them, split the amount to be converted into hundreds, tens, units and decimals and look up each of these separately; then add the answers for each.

For example, to convert 174 inches into millimetres, look up the figures for 100 inches then for 70 and then 4, and add all these together. 100 inches = 2500 mm; 70 inches = 1750 mm;

4 inches = 100 mm; 2500 + 1750 + 100 = 4350 mm. Therefore, 174 inches = 4350 mm. Before these tables are used to convert parts of a whole, it will be necessary to change the amount to be converted, if it is expressed as a vulgar fraction, into a decimal fraction, e.g. $\frac{1}{5}$ inch = 0·2.

TABLE 1

Millimetres	Inches	Inches	Millimetres
1000	40	100	2500
900	36	90	2250
800	32	80	2000
700	28	70	1750
600	24	60	1500
500	20	50	1250
400	16	40	1000
300	12	30	750
200	8	20	500
100	4	10	250
90	3·6	9	225
80	3·2	8	200
70	2·8	7	175
60	2·4	6	150
50	2·0	5	125
40	1·6	4	100
30	1·2	3	75
20	0·8	2	50
10	0·4	1	25
9	0·36	0·9	22·5
8	0·32	0·8	20
7	0·28	0·7	17·5
6	0·24	0·6	15
5	0·2	0·5	12·5
4	0·16	0·4	10
3	0·12	0·3	7·5
2	0·08	0·2	5
1	0·04	0·1	2·5

Exercises

1. Convert each of the following to inches:

(a) 946 mm   (b) 33 mm   (c) 128 mm
(d) 37 mm   (e) 85 mm   (f) 1263 mm

(*g*) 21 mm   (*h*) 14 mm   (*i*) 178 mm

2. Convert each of the following to millimetres:

(*a*) 42 in   (*b*) 88 in   (*c*) 1¾ in   (*d*) 22½ in   (*e*) 38 in
(*f*) 2·9 in   (*g*) 14·6 in   (*h*) 56·8 in   (*i*) 72 in

3. A certain film star's measurements are 36, 22, 35. How might this be expressed in France?

TABLE 2

Kilograms	Pounds		Pounds	Kilograms
100	220		100	45·4
90	198		90	40·9
80	176		80	36·3
70	154		70	31·8
60	132		60	27·2
50	110		50	22·7
40	88		40	18·2
30	66		30	13·6
20	44		20	9·1
10	22		10	4·5
9	19·8		9	4·1
8	17·6		8	3·6
7	15·4		7	3·2
6	13·2		6	2·7
5	11		5	2·3
4	8·8		4	1·8
3	6·6		3	1·4
2	4·4		2	0·9
1	2·2		1	0·45

4. Convert the following to pounds:

(*a*) 65 kg   (*b*) 132 kg   (*c*) 48 kg   (*d*) 21 kg   (*e*) 106 kg
(*f*) 33 kg   (*g*) 76 kg   (*h*) 16 kg   (*i*) 52 kg

5. Convert the following to kilograms:

(*a*) 74 lb   (*b*) 153 lb   (*c*) 33 lb   (*d*) 92 lb   (*e*) 74 lb
(*f*) 39 lb   (*g*) 66 lb   (*h*) 68 lb   (*i*) 21 lb

6. The following are the weights of patients. Convert them to metric units:

(*a*) 7 st 12 lb   (*b*) 8 st 2 lb   (*c*) 10 st 6 lb   (*d*) 14 st
(*e*) 13 st 7 lb   (*f*) 15 st

7. A patient is told he is 1 st 4 lb overweight. How much is this in kilograms?

8. The doctor orders 4 mg per kg of body weight to be given. If the patient weighs 156 lb, how much drug is he given in mg?

TABLE 3

Millilitres	Fl. Ounces	Fl. Ounces	Millilitres
1000	35	10	285
900	31·5	9	257
800	28	8	228
700	24·5	7	200
600	21	6	172
500	17·5	5	143
400	14	4	114
300	10·5	3	86
200	7	2	57
100	3·5	1	28
90	3·1	0·9	26
80	2·8	0·8	23
70	2·5	0·7	20
60	2·1	0·6	17
50	1·8	0·5	14
40	1·4	0·4	11
30	1·1	0·3	9
20	0·7	0·2	6
10	0·35	0·1	3

9. Convert the following to fluid ounces:
(a) 530 ml (b) 220 ml (c) 1910 ml (d) 830 ml (e) 640 ml
(f) 320 ml (g) 750 ml (h) 550 ml (i) 470 ml

10. Convert the following to millilitres:
(a) 53 fl oz (b) 28 fl oz (c) 33 fl oz (d) 4·6 fl oz
(e) 15 fl oz (f) 4·1 fl oz (g) 32 fl oz (h) 9·6 fl oz
(i) 83 fl oz

10
Percentages

IF THE words 'per cent' are translated, they mean 'per hundred' for which the symbol '%' is often used. The uncertainty that may arise in the mind when the words per cent are met with can usually be removed if it is remembered that they mean simply 'in each hundred' or 'in every hundred'. Thus, if it is said that 52% of the English population is female it means that fifty-two people *in every hundred* are female.

85% of the world's population have Rhesus positive blood.

30% of urban children are Mantoux positive by the age of 15 years.

This method is so concise and convenient that it is one of the favourite tools of the statistician. Indeed it is becoming so common, particularly in American semi-scientific accounts, that it is being used increasingly as a joke by stage comedians!

One of the greatest advantages of the percentage system is that it gives people a small, easily managed figure that can be used as a yardstick for making comparisons, where the actual figures would convey little or nothing. For example, if we take the unemployment figures for the United Kingdom in the early 1960s we see that approximately 300,000 people were unemployed in a population of about 40 million. 300,000 is approximately $\frac{3}{4}$% of that number. In the summer of 1971 the number of unemployed people increased to nearly 1 million in a population that has increased to over 50 million. Thus the percentage has increased to nearly 2%. In a case such as this the use of percentages permits direct comparisons to be made.

The greatest use made of percentages in the everyday work of a nurse is in strengths of liquid solutions. We are all conversant with such things as sodium citrate $2\frac{1}{2}\%$, cocaine 1%, surgical spirit 70%, chloroxylerol 20% and others. In all such cases, the actual quantities used may be of little

100 oz = $2\frac{1}{2}$ oz + $97\frac{1}{2}$ oz
Powder Water
(Solution of $2\frac{1}{2}$ oz)

10 Grammes = 0·1 +. 9·9
Gramme Grammes
powder water
(Solution of 0·1 gramme)

1 litre = 200 ml + 800 ml
liquid water

account. The strength is what matters, and whether one has 1 millilitre or 1 litre of a 1% solution, it remains a 1% solution. To find out exactly how much of a particular substance, the 'active principle', is present is the work of a moment if the strength is known, and also the total quantity one is dealing with. For instance, to find out how much pure chloroxylerol is present in a litre of solution of 5% strength, one says to oneself: 'In a 5% solution there are 5 parts of pure chloroxylerol in every 100 parts of solution. If there were 100 litres of solution it would contain 5 litres of chloroxylerol. If there were 100 millilitres it would contain 5 millilitres. Therefore I can say that 5-hundredths ($\frac{5}{100}$) of any quantity of 5% solution will be the amount of pure substance contained in that particular quantity. Hence $\frac{5}{100}$ of a litre is the amount of pure chloroxylerol in 1 litre of 5% strength.'

$\frac{5}{100}$ of a litre is an unwieldy measure. It is far better to express it in millilitres. This involves a little arithmetic and one continues thus: 'There are 1000 millilitres in a litre. Therefore $\frac{5}{100}$ of a litre is 50 millilitres.

$$\frac{5}{\underset{1}{100}} \times \overset{10}{1000} = 50.$$

Therefore, in every litre of 5% chloroxylerol there are 50 millilitres of pure chloroxylerol.

By similar reasoning one can work out such questions as, 'How much pure substance is required to make a particular quantity of solution of a particular strength, or how much can be made with a certain quantity?'

We have seen enough of fractions and decimals to know that they are interchangeable. So too with percentages. If 10% represents 10 parts in 100 parts it is the same thing as the fraction $\frac{10}{100}$, which in its simplest terms is $\frac{1}{10}$. This in its turn, is the same as 0·1.

Similarly 3% is the same as $\frac{3}{100}$ or 0·03

17% is the same as $\frac{17}{100}$ or 0·17

14·8% is the same as $\frac{14·8}{100}$ or 0·148

Therefore it is true to say that **any percentage figure can be written in fractional form by placing the percentage figure down as the numerator with 100 as the denominator.** In other words —divide the percentage figure by 100.

The converse of this is that **any fraction can be written as a percentage figure by multiplying the fraction by 100.**

$$\tfrac{3}{4} = \tfrac{3}{4} \times 100 \text{ per cent.}$$
$$= \tfrac{300}{4}$$
$$= 75\%$$

The rules for converting decimals to percentages and *vice versa* are similar. **Any percentage figure can be written in decimal form by dividing the figure by 100.**

$$75\% = 75 \div 100 = 0{\cdot}75$$

Conversely, **Any decimal fraction can be written in percentage form by multiplying the decimal by 100.**

$$0{\cdot}25 = 0{\cdot}25 \times 100 \text{ per cent} = 25\%$$

Expressing things in percentage form is a convenient and short form which applies to any quantity which, expressed in actual concrete units, would have to be different in each individual case. For instance, if one determines that one will save some money each month, it is a much better idea to decide that a certain percentage shall be banked, say 5% or 10%, than to fix on a definite quantity, say £2. In this way the amount saved will vary with the income each month. If there have been a lot of deductions leaving less than is usual, one is faced with banking a smaller amount and one's resolve is not embarrassed by having to deduct yet another £2 from a slim income. On the other hand, when one's salary is swollen with bonus, income tax rebate or emoluments for holiday periods, one has the satisfaction of seeing a larger quantity than £2 tucked safely away. The concrete amount varies from month to month but still remains 5% whether it is on £10 or £10 million.

To work out the concrete sums is but the work of a few

moments. Simply multiply the amount by the percentage figure and divide by 100.

Example 1: If it has been agreed that 5% of the beds available in a small town will be kept vacant for sudden emergency, how many beds are so reserved if there is a total bed list of 400?

Multiplying the total beds available by the percentage figure and dividing by 100 gives us this expression:

$$\frac{400 \times 5}{100} = 20$$

Therefore there are 20 beds reserved.

Example 2: (i) How much chlorhexidine in its pure state is required to make 2 gallons of 10% solution?

2 gallons multiplied by 1 and divided by 100

$$= \frac{320 \text{ fl oz} \times 1}{100} = 3 \cdot 2 \text{ fl oz}$$

$$= 3 \cdot 2 \text{ fl oz of pure chlorhexidine in 2 gallons.}$$

(ii) How much chlorhexidine in its pure state is required to make 9 litres of 1% solution.

$$\frac{9 \times 1}{100} = \frac{9}{100} = 0 \cdot 09 \text{ litre}$$

$0 \cdot 09$ litre $= 0 \cdot 9$ decilitres $= 9 \cdot 0$ centilitres $= 90 \cdot 0$ millilitres.

Example 3: If simple interest is paid by a loan club at the rate of $2\frac{1}{2}$% per annum how much interest is paid on £45 in 2 years?

Interest in 1 year is $\dfrac{£45 \times 2\frac{1}{2}}{100}$

In 2 years it is twice this

$$= \frac{£45 \times 2\frac{1}{2} \times 2}{100}$$

$$= £45 \times \tfrac{5}{2} \times 2 \times \tfrac{1}{100} = £\tfrac{9}{4}$$

$$= £2\tfrac{1}{4} = £2 \cdot 25$$

Exercises

1. Convert each of the following percentage figures to (i) fractions, and (ii) decimals:

(a) 1%   (b) 10%   (c) 15%   (d) 20%

(e) 40%   (f) 50%   (g) 75%   (h) 90%

2. Convert each of the following fractions to percentage figures:

(a) $\frac{1}{100}$ (b) $\frac{1}{20}$ (c) $\frac{6}{25}$ (d) $\frac{7}{20}$

(e) $\frac{81}{900}$ (f) $\frac{24}{25}$ (g) $\frac{3}{4}$ (h) $\frac{7}{8}$

3. Rewrite each of the following decimals as percentages:

(a) 0·3   (b) 0·75   (c) 0·42   (d) 0·01

(e) 0·66   (f) 0·25   (g) 0·305   (h) 0·393

4. If 25% of a class of 32 nurses have a negative reaction to the Heaf test, how many should receive B.C.G.?

5. How much pure ammonia is in a bottle containing 300 ml of Strong Ammonia Solution if it is a 40% solution?

6. How much pure chloroxylerol is required to make 2 litres of 10% dilution?

7. A nurse gets 40 marks out of 60 in a test. Express this as a percentage.

8. If 25% of the proceeds from a sale of work is sent to the Royal College of Nursing how much is sent if the sale nets £84·52?

9. If 15% of the patients in a hospital of 400 are under 21 years of age how many adults are there?

10. Calculate the superannuation payable to a retiring nurse if she is to get 40% of her salary annually and has been getting £1650 per annum.

11
Arithmetic and the body fluids

THERE are about 47 litres of water in the body of an adult person weighing 70 kg—between 60% and 70% of his total weight. At first this may seem to be a great deal of water, but when one considers the vast number of chemical changes that are happening in every part of the body, almost all of which depend on water, the wonder is not that there is so much but that the body is able to manage with so little. This is because this water is constantly on the move: into and out of the cells; into the digestive tract, and then back into the blood for use elsewhere; carrying wastes into the kidneys, leaving them there and passing back into the blood again for other tasks; into the cerebrospinal fluid, and out again; and so on. Indeed, life itself depends on this constant movement of water. Every cell needs a regular supply of raw materials to perform its functions, and these can reach the cells only when dissolved in water. Each cell must get rid of its waste substances and its manufactured products, and these also can be transported only when dissolved in water.

For convenience the 47 litres of water in the body may be considered as divided into two major lots; that inside the cells is called the intracellular fluid, and there is about 34 litres of this; outside the cells are about 10 litres of extracellular fluid. These are the two major divisions. In addition there are about 3 litres of water in the blood and 100 to 150 ml in the cerebrospinal fluid.

For these quantities to remain fairly constant, losses from the body must be balanced by intake, and in healthy people this occurs. Excessive consumption of fluids is quickly followed by increased output, and when the output causes the total quantities to fall below a certain level thirst is experienced and the loss is made good by drinking. In illness the balance is often upset and one of the major tasks of the nurse is to keep accurate records of intake and output and to try to balance these each day. In Chapter 17 the methods used to keep these records is explained.

Inside the body we find that the blood is the transport system which carries water to and from the places where it is needed. In the digestive system over 5 litres of water are secreted each day and almost all of this is reabsorbed back into the blood. About 1500 ml of saliva, 2500 ml of gastric juice, 700 ml of pancreatic juice, 500 ml bile and about 200 ml of intestinal juice are needed for the digestion and absorption of food. In order to get rid of the waste products dissolved in the blood, very large amounts of water are filtered out of it each day. About 137 litres of water pass from the blood into the kidney tubules, but almost all of this is taken back into the blood, and only about 1000 to 1500 ml leave the body each day in the form of urine. Everywhere we find the same sort of cycle, from blood to tissue fluid, from tissue fluid into the cells, and then back again to the blood via the tissue fluid or the lymph. Hence very little water is lost compared with the huge quantities that are used. Losses occur mainly in urine, about 1000 to 1500 ml; in sweat, the amount of which is very variable but is at least 500 ml a day; from the lungs, also variable and depending on the humidity of the external air, about 400 ml; and a little in faeces and in tears.

Blood

Blood is an extremely complex liquid consisting of 55% plasma and 45% cells. Many substances are dissolved in the plasma and as long as a person remains healthy the concentrations of these vary very little. During illness changes may occur and it is common in hospitals nowadays for specimens of blood to be taken from patients so that the laboratory staff can analyse them and estimate the quantities of solutes that are present. In this way diagnoses can be made or confirmed, treatment can be regulated and the progress that the patient is making can be checked.

One of the common tests carried out is to determine the amount of glucose in the blood. This is normally between 80 and 120 mg per 100 ml, but in diabetes mellitus it is greater. Insulin is therefore injected to reduce the figure, but there is no standard dose suitable to all diabetics. Each patient has to be stabilized on a daily dosage peculiar to his own condition and this may involve repeated examinations of the blood. If too much insulin is given the level of glucose in the blood falls dangerously low, while not enough insulin allows a gradual accumulation of glucose until it reaches dangerously high levels. Attention must be paid to the diet at the same time as insulin dosage is being established, so that the carbohydrates from which glucose is derived are kept at a constant daily intake. To balance the two, and yet to provide a nourishing and interesting diet, is a fascinating problem involving arithmetic, nutrition, dietetics and biochemistry.

Another test often performed is one designed to discover the amount of blood urea. Normally there is between 20 to 40 mg in each 100 ml of blood. Urea is a waste product derived from the metabolism of proteins and the kidneys are responsible for its removal from the blood. In kidney disease the ability to excrete urea and other protein wastes is impaired and the amount of damaged kidney tissue can be estimated by measuring the amount of urea in the blood.

Blood Clotting

The ability of blood to coagulate, or clot, is not fully understood. The process involves the interaction of several substances, some of which have not yet been isolated and identified but are nevertheless thought to be present. One of the known substances needed is an enzyme called thrombin. It is not present as such in blood except as prothrombin, an inactive forerunner of thrombin. During the clotting process prothrombin is turned into thrombin, which then acts on fibrinogen to make fibres of fibrin which entrap the blood cells to form the jelly-like clot. If there is insufficient prothrombin the time needed to form a clot is extended and severe haemorrhage may occur in the meantime.

Normally there are about 40 mg of prothrombin in each 100 ml of plasma. This figure is maintained by new prothrombin which is made in the liver, but only if there is an adequate supply of vitamin K. If there is insufficient vitamin K the blood level of prothrombin falls and then there is a danger that haemorrhage will occur. This is seen in people with obstructive jaundice or other conditions where no bile is passing into the intestines. It occurs in these cases because bile is necessary for the absorption of vitamin K. A blood test soon shows when the prothrombin level has fallen and, from this, the amount of vitamin K that will have to be injected. In some forms of hepatitis the liver cells lose their ability to make prothombin even though there is a plentiful supply of vitamin K. The efficiency of the liver can be determined by comparing the amounts of prothrombin before and after injections of vitamin K.

In certain diseases the blood may clot inside a blood vessel. This is called thrombosis and the clot is called a thrombus. In the treatment of such conditions drugs called anticoagulants are used. Two of these, dicoumarol and phenindione (Dindevan), interfere with the formation of prothrombin and so render the blood less liable to clotting. These drugs are dangerous and their use is controlled by a careful watch on the blood level of prothrombin.

Haemoglobin

Oxygen is needed by every cell in the body tissues. It is carried to them in the red cells of the blood, which are filled with a protein substance called haemoglobin. The normal quantity of haemoglobin is about 13 to 16 g per 100 ml of blood, 1 gramme of haemoglobin combines with 1·34 ml of oxygen. Thus the amount of haemoglobin gives a good guide to the oxygen-carrying capacity. In many diseases the level of haemoglobin falls. This may or may not be accompanied by a fall in the number of red cells, depending on what is causing the anaemia. As the cause is treated the amount of haemoglobin rises to normal and may exceed this, so checks are carried out throughout the treatment.

It is usual to give the figure for haemoglobin as a percentage; 14·8 g of haemoglobin in 100 ml of blood is assumed to be the normal. Hence a haemoglobin of 100% represents 14·8 g per 100 ml; 120% is 17·76 g per 100 ml, 60% is 8·88 g per 100 ml, and so on.

Blood Cells

When a specimen of blood is taken for estimation of red and white cell content, the laboratory technician is faced with a long and intricate task. The normal average red cell content of blood is 5 to 6 million per cubic millimetre (5 to 6 $\times$ 10^6/mm^3); white cells average 6000 to 10,000/mm^3, and platelets 200,000 to 500,000/mm^3. If the laboratory technician had actually to count these in a cubic millimetre the task would be Herculean indeed. You might like to calculate how long it would take you to count up to five million, without stopping, at the rate of 20 per second. It works out at somewhere near 70 hr! From this it is obvious that a simple method had to be devised for counting cells in blood.

The method involves diluting the blood to a strength of 1 in 200 with a special diluting liquid that will not damage the cells in any way. The red cells present in $\frac{1}{50}$ of a cubic millimetre are counted and the result is multiplied by 50 and 200 to give the number present in 1 mm^3. The figure is correct within 10,000 cells provided the actual counting has been done carefully.

White cell counts are done in a similar fashion but the blood is first diluted to a strength of 1 in 20. The diluting fluid is of such a nature that the red cells present are destroyed but the white cells are untouched. This makes counting a simpler task. The counting chamber is marked out in large squares for white cell counts, each large square having an area of 1 square millimetre. The volume of dilute blood appearing over one of these large squares is $1 \times \frac{1}{10}$ mm^3. Hence the number of white cells appearing within the boundaries of one large square is the number present in 0·1 mm^3 of blood diluted to a strength of 1 in 20. This number has only to be multiplied by 200 (10 and 20) to give the number of white cells in 1 mm^3 of pure blood. For greater accuracy more large squares are used than just one. Four is a convenient number and the cells counted are multiplied by 50 to give the final figure.

Differentiating between the different types of white cells is a skill that comes only from experience, but what the expert discovers when he looks down his microscope can be turned into percentage figures by anyone who can multiply and divide.

As all these cells fluctuate rather widely it is usual to express them in percentage figures of the total number.

Urine

Another source of material for laboratory investigation is urine. Like blood, this is a solution of many substances and the amounts of solutes can be measured. The average composition is: water, 96%; urea, 2%; various salts, chiefly sodium chloride, 2%.

In health the amount of urine excreted varies between 500 and 2000 ml, and the quantity depends on intake, sweating, external temperature and exercise. Increased output occurs whenever the amount of fluid consumed is increased or when there is a drop in the temperature of the environment. In some diseases there is an increase in output, as in diabetes mellitus. In this condition increased quantities of water are needed to excrete the glucose in solution. In the condition called diabetes insipidus there is a large output because the hormone, vasopressin, is lacking. This hormone encourages the reabsorption of water in the renal tubules. Shortage of it allows an extra large proportion of the water in the body to be discharged as urine. Thirst is a symptom.

Diuretics are drugs which encourage the output of urine. In some conditions where oedema occurs such drugs are used extensively. Some of them, especially the mercurial diuretics, can damage the kidney and must be used with care. Caffeine, which is present in tea and coffee, has a diuretic effect.

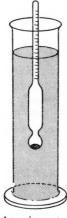

An urinometer

The specific gravity of urine is the weight of a certain quantity of urine compared with the weight of an equal volume of water. It reflects the quantity of dissolved matter in the urine; the greater the quantity of solute the higher the specific gravity, and *vice versa*. Specific gravities are usually expressed as a comparison with the weight of 1 ml of water, which is 1 gramme; but in urine analysis it is more convenient to use the weight of 1 litre of water, which is 1000 g. So a specific gravity of urine of 1025 indicates that there are 25 g of solutes in each litre.

It would be possible to find the specific gravity of urine by actually weighing a specimen; but it is far more convenient to use an instrument called a urinometer. This is a special form of hydrometer adapted for use in urine; and the stem is graduated so that specific gravities can be read off directly. The urinometer is immersed in the urine and should not touch the containing vessel at any point. When the urinometer comes to rest the depth to which it has sunk is noted and the figure on the scale which is level with the surface of the urine is the specific gravity of that specimen. Most urinometers are graduated from 0 at the top to 50 at the base of the stem. Whatever figure is read off is added to 1000 to give the final reading.

In health the specific gravity of urine usually varies between 1010 and 1030. As the total amount of waste matter to be excreted in 24 hr is fairly constant in normal healthy people, this variation in specific gravity is caused by the variable amounts of water and other liquids taken. The most concentrated specimen is usually that passed on rising in the morning.

When the kidney is damaged it loses its ability to concentrate urine, and the specific gravity remains constant irrespective of the variations in the amount of fluid consumed. The figure is often constant at about 1010 to 1012. It is easy to see how this happens. A normal healthy kidney can pack all the waste products passing through it into whatever water is available, whereas a diseased kidney cannot do so. If there is only a little water available the diseased kidney will get rid of some of the waste, but any that is left over has to return to the general circulation. If there is plenty of water the diseased kidney is able to excrete its normal quota and is able to get rid of some of the backlog as well. So, no matter what the conditions may be, the specific gravity remains the same. Nurses are usually entrusted with the determination of specific gravity and they should make every effort to see that it is done accurately.

Sometimes it happens that a specimen is insufficient in quantity for the urinometer to float without touching the bottom of the jar. When this happens the quantity of urine should be measured carefully and an exactly equal quantity of water added. When the figure on the stem of the urinometer is read it should be doubled. If adding an equal quantity of water is insufficient, twice the quantity can be added but then when the specific gravity of the mixture is taken the figure should be trebled to give the correct reading. For instance, let us say that the patient can provide only 60 ml of urine. If we then add 60 ml of water and find the urinometer reading is 06 the specific gravity of the specimen is 1012. If we had added 120 ml of water we would have found the reading to be 04 for a specific gravity of 1012.

Cerebrospinal Fluid

Around the brain and spinal cord and in the ventricles of the brain and the central canal of the cord there is a liquid called the cerebrospinal fluid (CSF). Examination of this fluid is an important clinical routine. It is a clear, colourless alkaline fluid with a specific gravity of 1005 to 1008. It contains much the same constituents as plasma, but without the plasma proteins; there are also significant differences in the concentration of the solutes.

There are about 100 to 150 ml of CSF. It is made from blood in the choroid plexuses of the brain ventricles and is reabsorbed into the capillaries of the arachnoid mater. How fast it is produced is not known, but when it is allowed to escape freely more than 500 ml a day is made.

The pressure that exists in the CSF depends on the position of the body; when lying flat it is sufficient to support 100 to 200 mm of water; in the erect position it is about double this figure. In many conditions, such as head injury, tumour of the brain or meningitis, the pressure is raised and the amounts of solute are altered. Specimens are usually taken by 'lumbar puncture', in which a needle is inserted into the fluid where it extends into a space below the end of the spinal cord.

Electrolytes

Many of the solutes in the various fluids of the body carry an electrical charge. They are electrolytes and contain *ions*, which are atoms that have lost or gained one or two electrons and have therefore become electrically charged. They can also partake in chemical changes.

Their ability to partake in chemical change depends not on their weight but on their electrical charge and so it is preferable to measure their chemical ability rather than their weight. The unit of chemical combining power is called the *milli-equivalent* and is defined as the combining power of 1 mg of hydrogen. Therefore the quantity of a chemical that has an equal combining power to that of 1 mg of hydrogen is 1 milli-equivalent. Hence, the following are all 1 milli-equivalents 1 mg hydrogen, 35 mg chloride, 20 mg calcium, 4,140 mg proteinate.

Expressing electrolytes in milli-equivalents saves a great deal of laborious calculation when it comes to administering fluids to patients who are suffering from imbalance of their electrolytes. The older method of expressing solutes in the form of so many milligrams per 100 ml of solution is gradually being replaced and we see more and more the symbol mEq/l meaning milli-equivalents per litre.

It is easy enough to convert mg/100 ml to mEq/l providing the valency and the atomic weight of the solute is known. This conversion is done with the formula:

$$\frac{mg/100 \text{ ml} \times 10 \times \text{valency}}{\text{atomic weight}} = mEq/l$$

but few people carry valencies and atomic weights around in their heads.

Electrolytes are of two kinds: those carrying negative charges and those carrying positive charges. Those carrying negative charges are called *anions* and those carrying positive charges are called *cations*. Cations can unite chemically with anions to form whole molecules and herein lies the secret of the balance of electrolytes in the body.

Taken as a whole the healthy body is electrically neutral. In other words such is the chemistry of the body that the number of cations and the number of anions are equal. Local imbalances are bound to occur but are soon corrected to keep the whole system stable. Imbalances probably occur in every disease, and in some diseases on a scale large enough to upset the normal activities of the cells. In some illnesses the imbalance may be so severe that death occurs very rapidly and great effort must be made to keep the electrolytes balanced.

In any condition where there is loss of body fluids there will also be loss of electrolytes and consequent upset in the delicate balance. In vomiting, diarrhoea, burns, haemorrhage and shock, gross imbalances are met with and the first consideration of the doctor is to correct them. The following table shows the important solutes found in tissue fluid and expressed in mEq/l in round figures for ease of memory:

Sodium	150
Chloride	100
Potassium	4
Carbon dioxide	30

Exercises

1. If a person's body contains 5 litres of blood and there are 5 million red cells in each cubic millimetre, how many red cells are there altogether?

2. From the answer to the previous question work out the total area that the red cells cover if each red cell has a surface area of 0·0001 mm^2 in square metres and converted to square yards (1 m^2 = $1\frac{1}{6}$ sq yd).

3. If 4% of the oxygen in inspired air is absorbed into the red cells with each breath, what is the total volume of oxygen absorbed in 1 minute if 500 cm³ of air are inspired 15 times per minute? (Air is 20% oxygen.)

4. From the following data work out the percentage of each type of white cell to the total number.

Total number per cubic millimetre	6000
Neutrophils	2400
Eosinophils	200
Basophils	100
Lymphocytes	2600
Monocytes	700

5. The number of red cells counted in $\frac{1}{50}$ cubic millimetre of blood diluted to 1 in 200 is 485. What is the number of red cells per cubic millimetre of pure blood?

6. Given that haemoglobin 100% represents 14·8 g per 100 ml, find how much haemoglobin there is when it is 40%, 66%, 80% and 105%.

12
Solutions

A SOLUTION occurs when any two substances are mixed together so intimately that their *molecules* are mingled in juxtaposition. Any two substances can form solutions provided that the mixing is on a molecular level, but only certain substances can mix together in this way. The commonest form of solution is that of a solid in a liquid, but soda water is a solution of water and carbon dioxide, i.e. a gas dissolved in a liquid, and many kinds of oil are soluble in alcohol, i.e. one liquid dissolved in another. Gases also may hold substances in solution, e.g. air may take up a certain amount of water and the mixture may be regarded as water dissolved in air.

Metal alloys are solutions of solids, although they are usually mixed while the solids are in liquid state. This is not always the case, however, and gold and lead laid together in thin sheets and subject to pressure will coalesce to form a metal alloy. Stirring sugar into tea gives us an everyday example of a solution of a solid in a liquid.

In hospitals the word 'solution' usually refers to a liquid, a liquid in which two liquids have been mixed together or one in which a solid has been dissolved in a liquid. The substance dissolved or the lesser quantity is referred to as the *solute* while the liquid in which the solute has been dissolved is called the *solvent*. Sometimes words other than solvent are used, such as diluent, vehicle or medium. Essentially they mean the same thing.

A good everyday example of a solution used in hospitals is saline. This is merely salty water. Salt is the solute and water is the solvent. Chlorhexidine lotion is a solution of chlorhexidine in water. Chlorhexidine is the solute and water is the solvent. (Spirit is used as the solvent for some purposes.) When one uses ether to remove grease from the skin one is using the solvent powers of ether. Ether is the solvent and the grease is the solute.

Almost always the solutions in hospitals use water as the solvent. When alcohol is used the solution is usually called a tincture. If the solvent is one that evaporates very quickly leaving the solute behind as a solid the solution may be called a collodion.

The nurse's duties very rarely include the making of solutions other than those with water as the solvent. Preparation of all others is normally undertaken by the pharmacist, who is trained especially for such work. So too with substances for injection. Anything that has to be injected must be prepared under the strictest aseptic precautions and it is better to have a special department with specially trained staff for such work. Although this is so, nurses frequently have to make up solutions such as penicillin, streptomycin, thiopentone and local anaesthetics, so it is necessary for them to know how to make specified strength solutions with a high degree of accuracy. Since this book is concerned merely with the arithmetic of such matters, stress has not been laid on the aseptic precautions that are essential to perfect nursing technique. Hence no such details are included here though a timely reminder has been sometimes added in parenthesis.

Very many solutions are used in hospitals and it is convenient to separate them under headings and categories.

1. Solutions for external application to the body, such as hexachlorophane, acriflavine, cetrimide, eusol.

2. Solutions for disinfection of substances to be used again, such as phenol, sudol.

3. Solutions for the disinfection of discharges and excreta which will be discarded, such as sudol.

4. Solutions for the sterilization of instruments, such as glutaraldehyde, formalin and chlorhexidine.

5. Solutions for application to mucous surfaces, such as cocaine, hydrogen peroxide, potassium permanganate, glycerin.

6. Solutions for intramuscular injection, such as strepto-mycin, penicillin.

The nurse may be called upon to make up such solutions and she *must* be able to do so accurately. Some solutions must be made from drugs of extreme potency, sometimes the solute is in powder or crystal or tablet form; sometimes the solvent is water but this may have to be distilled water or pyrogen-free sterile water. For external soaks, baths, mouth-washes and disinfectants ordinary tap water is usually suitable. For silver nitrate solutions distilled water is necessary. For all solutions for injection pyrogen-free sterile water is required, together with an aseptic technique.

All this needs an understanding of the terminology and the arithmetic of solutions before a nurse can proceed with confidence. Two abbreviations may cause some confusion at first. They are 'v/v solution' and 'w/v solution'.

v/v solutions are those in which the amount of solute and the amount of the solvent can both be measured in volume units. For instance cetrimide is a liquid and a measure of capacity is used to describe the quantity. Water can be similarly measured so that a solution of cetrimide can readily be made with millilitre and litre measures.

w/v solutions are those in which the solute is a solid and must be measured in *weight* units. The solvent is measured in *volume* units but for the calculation of the strength the volume units of the solvent are converted into weight units. The strength is then calculated with both substances expressed in *weight* units. Essentially that is all there is to the calculation of w/v solutions and it is no more difficult than the calculation of v/v solution strengths. The relationship between volume and weight in the metric system is helpful as one millilitre of

water weighs one gramme. A litre of water weighs one kilogram, etc.

Exercises

1. Using a millilitre measure pour out 5 millilitres of
pure carbolic acid. Transfer this to a larger measure. Add a
little water to the small measure to take up the remaining
carbolic acid and add this to the large measure. Add water
until there is a total of 400 millilitres. You have then made a
v/v solution of carbolic acid. The strength is 5 ml in 400 ml, or
1 in 80.

2. Using a millilitre measure pour 20 ml of red ink.
Empty this into a litre measure. Add water to the large
measure to make a total of 1 litre. You have now made a
v/v solution of red ink. The strength is 20 ml in 1 litre; this is
1 in 50.

3. Add 4 g of salt to 300 ml of water. One millilitre weighs
1 g, therefore 300 ml weighs 300 g. The weight of the solution is 300 g + 4 g = 304 g. 4 g of salt is 304 g = 1 g in 76 g.
You have now made a w/v solution.

Strengths of solutions

Ratio Strengths

The strength of a solution can be expressed in three ways,
ratio strength, percentage strength and dose strength. In the
foregoing three exercises ratio strength has been used—one
part in so many parts. To find the ratio strength of a solution
the *total quantity of the solution* is divided by the *amount of
solute* and the answer is expressed as one in whatever the
figure may be. Both the quantities must be in the same units
to find the strength. It does not matter what units are used
provided they are the same for solute and total quantity.

Therefore, the rules for finding ratio strength of a solution are thus:

(1) Find the quantity of solute.
(2) Find the total quantity of solution in the same units.
(3) Divide the larger quantity by the smaller.
(4) Express the answer as one in this quotient.

Actually the answer can be written down in three ways. It can be written as 'one in something' which is the most expressive way, or in true ratio form with a colon between the two numbers, e.g. 1:20, 1:40, etc., or in simple fractional form, e.g. $\frac{1}{20}$, $\frac{1}{40}$, etc.

Example 1: Find the ratio strength of a solution in which 7 ml of pure substance have been added to 203 ml of water.

Quantity of solute $= 7$ ml
Total quantity of solution $= 203$ ml of water $+ 7$ ml solute
$= 210$ ml
$210 \div 7 = 30$
∴ Strength is 1 in 30.

This strength can also be written 1:30 or $\frac{1}{30}$.

Example 2: Find the ratio strength when 10 fl oz of a substance are made up to 2 gal with water.

Amount of solute $= 10$ fl oz
Total amount of solution $= 2$ gal $= 16$ pt
$= 320$ fl oz
$320 \div 10 = 32$
∴ the strength is 1 in 32 (1:32, $\frac{1}{32}$).

Note that in *Example 1* it was necessary to find the total quantity by adding the amount of solute and the amount of solvent whereas in *Example 2* the wording of the question made it clear that there was a total of 2 gal. All such questions must be read very carefully to make sure whether the quantity of solvent is mentioned or the total quantity of solution.

Ratio strengths are perfect examples of fractions. If you

turn back to pages 12 and 13 you will read that the denominator of a fraction expresses the total number of parts available and the numerator expresses the number of parts to be considered in any particular instance. Take the ratio strength 1 in 60 as an example. Put into fractional form $\frac{1}{60}$ it tells us that there are 60 parts altogether, the denominator, and that 1 part, the numerator, is pure drug, In all ratio strengths the amount of pure drug is expressed as 1 part while the total quantity varies, 10 parts, 20 parts, 1000 parts, etc.

Percentage Strengths

Quite frequently strength is expressed as a percentage instead of a ratio. This has been explained in Chapter 10 but a little application of that chapter is in order in this particular context. To find the percentage strength of a solution divide the amount of solute by the total quantity of solution and multiply by 100. As usual the amounts of solute and solution must be in the same units. Note too that once again the total quantity of solution is required and not merely the amount of solvent.

If the strength of a solution is already expressed in ratio form it can be turned into percentage form by expressing the ratio as a fraction and multiplying it by 100. Conversely, to change percentage strength to ratio strength write down the percentage figure as a fraction (with 100 as the denominator) and divide the denominator by the numerator in the margin. The quotient gives the ratio strength.

Example 1: What is the percentage strength when 1 fl oz of disinfectant concentrate is made up to 4 pints with water?

Amount of solute $= 1$ fl oz

Total amount of solution $= 80$ fl oz

∴ Percentage strength $= \frac{1}{80} \times 100 = \frac{10}{8} = 1\frac{1}{4}\%$

Example 2: What is the percentage strength when 3 g of silver nitrate is dissolved in 200 ml of water (distilled)?

(This is a w/v solution so both items must be expressed in weight units.)

$$\text{Amount of solute} = 3 \text{ g}$$
$$\text{Total amount of solution} = 200 \text{ ml}$$
$$200 \text{ ml weighs } 200 \text{ g}$$

$$\therefore \text{ Percentage strength} = \frac{3}{200} \times 100$$

$$= \frac{3}{2} \times 1 = 1\tfrac{1}{2}$$

This is expressed as $1\tfrac{1}{2}\%$ or $1\cdot 5\%$.

Example 3: If you are told that the sodium hypochlorite you are using is 1 in 80 what percentage strength would this be?

$$\text{Ratio strength} = 1 \text{ in } 80$$
$$\therefore \text{ Percentage strength} = \tfrac{1}{80} \times 100$$
$$= \frac{5}{4}\%$$
$$= 1\tfrac{1}{4}\%$$

Example 4: Express 20% as a ratio strength.

$$\text{Percentage strength} = 20$$
$$\therefore \text{Ratio strength } \tfrac{20}{100} = \tfrac{1}{5}$$
$$= 1 \text{ in } 5.$$

Dose strength

Stating the strengths of a solution in its dose strength is an extremely simple and easy-to-understand method. A certain quantity of drug is dissolved in a certain quantity of solvent and this is stated on the label. Insulin is probably the best example. The strength is stated as so many units per ml. 10, 20, 40 and 80 units per ml are the usual strengths. (U10, U20, U40 and U80 is the conventional method of stating this for insulin.) Many of the antibiotics are similarly expressed in dose strength, penicillin 100,000 units per ml, streptomycin 1 g in 2 ml, etc.

The usual problem with such drugs is to calculate the amount of solution to be given to ensure a certain quantity of drug. This is very simple arithmetic but accuracy is so important that it is worth while working through many theoretical examples.

Example 1: A diabetic is to receive 20 units of soluble insulin at 08.00 hours. What quantity will be given from a stock of U40 (40 units per ml)?

> 40 units in 1 ml
> ∴ 1 unit in $\frac{1}{40}$ ml
> ∴ 20 units in $\frac{1}{40} \times 20$ ml $= \frac{20}{40} = \frac{1}{2}$ ml
> ∴ Amount to be given is 0·5 ml

Example 2: How would you give a patient 60 units of insulin from U80 strength?

> 80 units in 1 ml
> ∴ 1 unit in $\frac{1}{80}$ ml
> ∴ 60 units in $\frac{1}{80} \times 60$ ml $= \frac{60}{80} = 0·75$ ml

Example 3: A patient is to have streptomycin 0·75 g daily. What quantity of solution will be given from a bottle labelled 2 g per ml?

> 2 g in 1 ml
> ∴ 1 g in $\frac{1}{2}$ ml
> ∴ $\frac{3}{4}$ g in $\frac{1}{2} \times \frac{3}{4}$ ml $= \frac{3}{8}$ ml
> ∴ 0·375 ml will be given each day

Example 4: How could you give a child 7·5 mg of morphine if the stock bottle is labelled 10 mg in 1 ml?

> 10 mg in 1 ml
> ∴ there is 1 mg in $\frac{1}{10}$ ml

$$\therefore \frac{1}{10} \times 7\frac{1}{2} = \frac{1 \times \overset{3}{\cancel{15}}}{\underset{2}{\cancel{10}} \times 2}$$

$$= \tfrac{3}{4} = 0.75$$

∴ I would give the child 0·75 ml.

Exercises

What quantity is required to give the correct amount of insulin in each of the following?

1.	32 units from U40
2.	16 ,, ,, U20
3.	12 ,, ,, U20
4.	60 ,, ,, U80
5.	6 ,, ,, U20
6.	6 ,, ,, U10
7.	44 ,, ,, U40
8.	15 ,, ,, U20

N.B. When the choice of strength to be used is left to the nurse she should choose one that will result in a quantity of less than 1 ml if it is possible. For instance, when a dose of 30 units is needed it is better to use U40 than U20.

Special insulin syringes are available that are graduated in units. This makes drawing up the required quantity incomparably easier but introduces a risk where different strengths are available. A U80 syringe is one in which the marked divisions are arranged so that there are 80 divisions to 1 ml. It is intended for use only with U80 insulin. Similarly a U20 syringe is graduated to show 20 units per ml and must not be used with any insulin other than U20 insulin. Only a very experienced nurse should use a syringe that is not graduated to match the particular strength insulin to be used and she should use it only in an emergency.

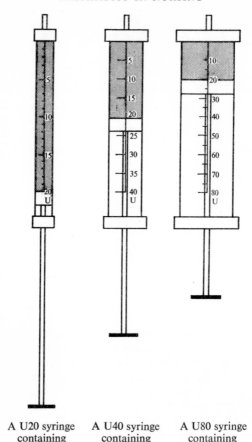

A U20 syringe
containing
20 units

A U40 syringe
containing
20 units

A U80 syringe
containing
20 units

Almost all mixtures for oral administration could be labelled giving the dose strength. All too frequently dispensers are content to label bottles with instructions only, 'Mist. Alb. Dose 30 ml' is the usual type of thing. This is a great pity as it robs the nurse of a chance to learn her pharmacology more thoroughly. How very much more informative it would be if the label read 'Mist. Alb.: Mag. Sulph. 8 g in 30 ml' or 'Mist. Pot. Brom.: Pot. Brom. 1 g in 15 ml Dose 15 ml'. All dispensaries should be urged to adopt this method, which is used in most of the leading hospitals.

A nurse can help herself in this matter. She should keep a booklet into which she writes the name of every mixture used in her ward. Alongside she should write the dose strength. Pharmacists are always agreeably surprised when nurses approach them with intelligent questions about dose strengths of mixtures and are usually quite keen to help.

Here is a list to start with. Find the dose strength and then work out the total quantity of drug dissolved in, say, a 240 ml bottle, and, to complete the record, the action of the drug.

Magnesium Sulphate Mixture (Mist. Alb.)

Kaolin and Morphine Mixture (Mist. Kaolin, et Morph.)

Liquid Extract of Cascara (Extr. Casc. Liq.)

Indomethacin Suspension

Potassium Bromide and Chloral Mixture (Mist. Pot. Brom. et Chloral.)

Potassium Bromide Mixture (Mist. Pot. Brom.)

Chloral Mixture (Mist. Chloral.)

Potassium Iodide Mixture (Mist. Pot. Iod.)

Ipecacuanha and Morphine Mixture (Mist. Ipecac. et Morph.)

Exercises

Calculate the ratio strength of each of the following:

 1.   Sudol 10 ml added to 390 ml water.
 2.   0·2 ml chlorhexidine in 1 litre of solution.
 3.   4 ml of cetrimide in 600 ml of solution.
 4.   300 mg of cocaine in 60 ml of water.

5. Five litres of solution containing 25 ml of sodium hypochlorite.
6. Silver nitrate 120 mg in 30 ml of water.

Convert each of the following to percentage strengths:

7. Stericol 1 in 80.
8. Chlorhexidine 1 in 1000.
9. Sudol 1 in 40.
10. Cetrimide 1 in 100.

Convert each of the following to ratio strengths:

11. Sodium citrate $2\frac{1}{2}\%$.
12. Magnesium sulphate 3%.
13. Cocaine 4%.
14. Sodium bicarbonate 1%.
15. Dextrose 5%.
16. Complete the blank spaces in the following chart:

Amount of of pure drug	Total amount of solution	Ratio strength	Percentage strength
(a)	100 ml		2%
(b)	2 pints	1 in 10	
(c) 3 ml			1%
(d) 15 ml		1 in 80	
(e) 4 ml			$\frac{5}{8}\%$
(f) 0·25 ml		1 in 1000	
(g)	30 litres		0·01%
(h)	40 ml		20%
(i) 2 ounces		1 in 20	
(j)	120 ml		$2\frac{1}{2}\%$
(k)	2 litres		$\frac{1}{2}\%$
(l)	$1\frac{1}{2}$ pints	1 in 60	
(m)	500 ml		0·2%
(n) 4 ml			$1\frac{1}{4}\%$
(o) 0·5 ml		1 in 80	

List three solutions used in your hospital for each of the following tasks. Give the ratio strength and the percentage strength. Work out how much pure drug you would need to make various appropriate quantities.

(1) Solutions for the disinfection of vomitus, urine, faeces, etc.
(2) Solutions used for the sterilization of surgical instruments.
(3) Solutions used for mouthwashes, rectal washout, gargles, etc.
(4) Solutions for irrigation of the stomach.
(5) Solutions used for bladder washout.
(6) Solutions used for the irrigation of wounds.
(7) Solutions used for eye drops.

13
Dilution of drugs and lotions

IT OFTEN occurs in wards, theatres and kitchens that a nurse requires to give a certain strength of drug or to use a certain strength of lotion, and all she has is something stronger. She has the right substance but it is too strong for her needs. We can all think of instances when such has been the case. We want to give morphine 15 mg and have only 20 mg, or we wish to use chlorhexidine 1 in 5000 when we are supplied with strength 1 in 1000.

Such problems are constantly arising and if the nurse cannot work out exactly how the dilution is to be performed, there is a risk that she will be tempted to go by guess-work. Getting it 'somewhere near' may be of little consequence when the dilution is required for the sterilization of contaminated items, but there is no room for guess-work where drugs are concerned, particularly when the drug is a dangerous one to be given in tiny fractions of a grain. We must be exact or else own up to our ignorance and hand over to someone who knows better. There is no disgrace in doing so, whereas proceeding in ignorance is criminal folly, and may cost a life.

When one follows the working of a few examples it is surprising how simple the process is. But one **must** follow the reasoning and work out plenty of theoretical examples so that when the situation arises in real life one can say to oneself, 'Ah! This is something I have mastered. I am on sure ground here', and can proceed with calm assurance.

Sometimes the problem is so simple that one can do the arithmetic mentally. As a general rule, however, it is better to take pencil and paper to make absolutely sure that there is no error.

For instance, in an example such as—How would you give morphine 7·5 mg if you have only ampoules of 15 mg.? It is obvious to one and all that 7·5 is half of 15 and that one should discard half the liquid and inject the other half. But if asked to give 7·5 mg when only ampoules of 20 mg are available, the answer may not be so obvious. We require some simple rule of thumb that will apply to all cases.

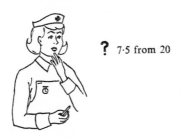

? 7·5 from 20

There is such a rule and stripped to its bare bones it states: **divide the strength you want by the strength you have.**

This should be memorized so that you can wake up in bed at three o'clock in the morning and repeat it without any doubt in your mind whatsoever.

Say to yourself whenever you have to deal with any of these problems, 'What strength do I **want**?' Write it down as a fraction.

Next you say to yourself, 'What strength have I **got**?' Write this alongside as another fraction and insert a division sign between the two.

From here on it is simple arithmetic. We have two fractions the first of which is going to be divided by the second. You will remember that the way to divide by a fraction is to turn it upside down and multiply by it. There will usually be some cancelling to do and the end result will be a fraction. This fraction is what you are after as it tells you how much of the substance you will need to take from the stock. For instance, if the resulting fraction is $\frac{1}{10}$ you will need to take $\frac{1}{10}$ of the final quantity from the stock and add to it sufficient water from the tap or from a bottle of sterile water to make it up to the quantity required.

Let us apply the rule to the first easy example that we mentioned before, that of giving 7·5 mg of morphine when only 15 mg ampoules are available. We already know the answer, so if our arithmetic comes out to anything different we had better examine the arithmetic.

The rule is—divide the strength you want by the strength you have.

$$\text{Strength wanted } = 7\cdot5 \text{ mg}$$
$$\text{Strength you have } = 15 \text{ mg in 1 ml}$$
$$7\tfrac{1}{2} \div 15 = \tfrac{15}{2} \div \tfrac{15}{1}$$
$$= \tfrac{15}{2} \times \tfrac{1}{15}$$
$$= \tfrac{1}{2}$$

Therefore half the quantity in the 15 mg ampoule will contain 7·5 mg. The other half is discarded.

Now let us have a look at the second example quoted. It said—how would you give 7·5 mg if you had only 20 mg ampoules.

Go about it in exactly the same way.

$$\text{Strength wanted } = 7\cdot5 \text{ mg}$$
$$\text{Strength supplied } = 20 \text{ mg in 1 ml}$$
$$7\tfrac{1}{2} \div 20 = \tfrac{15}{2} \div \tfrac{20}{1}$$
$$= \frac{\overset{3}{15}}{2} \times \frac{1}{\underset{4}{20}}$$
$$= \tfrac{3}{8}$$

Therefore three-eighths of 1 ml will contain 7·6 mg. The remaining $\frac{5}{8}$ are discarded.

In some instances the amounts to be dealt with are very small quantities. The rule applies equally well.

How can 400 microgrammes (μg) of atropine be given if the ward stock carries only ampoules of 600 μg of atropine?

$$\text{Strength wanted} = 400 \ \mu\text{g}$$
$$\text{Strength supplied} = 600 \ \mu\text{g in 1 ml}$$
$$400 \div 600 = \frac{400}{600} = \tfrac{2}{3} \ \text{ml}$$

Therefore $\tfrac{2}{3}$ ml contain the required dose, the remaining $\tfrac{1}{3}$ is discarded.

Another example with lotions.

How would you prepare from a stock bottle of chlorhexidine of strength 1 in 500, a litre of lotion of strength 1 in 2500?

$$\text{Strength wanted} = 1/2500$$
$$\text{Stock strength} = 1/500$$
$$\frac{1}{2500} \div \frac{1}{500}$$
$$= \frac{1}{2500} \times \frac{500}{1}$$
$$= \tfrac{5}{25}$$
$$= \tfrac{1}{5}$$

Therefore $\tfrac{1}{5}$ of 1 litre is taken from the stock bottle = $\tfrac{1}{5}$ of 1000 ml = 200 ml and the litre is made up by adding tap water.

When dealing with percentage solutions, the task becomes extremely simple because fractions need not enter into the calculation at all. The rule of dividing the strength required by the strength you have still holds.

For instance—How much chloroxylenol 10% is required to make 1 litre of 1% solution?

$$\text{Strength wanted} = 1\%$$
$$\text{Strength of stock} = 10\%$$
$$1 \div 10$$
$$= \tfrac{1}{10}$$

Therefore you will need $\tfrac{1}{10}$ of 1 litre from the 10% bottle which is 100 ml.

Children's Doses

The doses of drugs given in pharmacopoeias are usually adult doses. Special doses for children are given only for certain drugs. There are two accepted rules for working out a suitable dose for a child from the adult dose, Young's rule and Fried's rule. Young's rule is suitable for children over 1 year of age and Fried's rule for children under 1 year.

Young's rule states that a suitable children's dose can be found by multiplying the adult dose by the child's age in *years* and dividing this figure by the age in years plus 12.

$$\text{Child's dose} = \frac{\text{Adult's dose} \times \text{child's age in years}}{\text{Child's age in years} + 12}$$

Example 1: How much morphine can be given to a child of 6 years if the adult dose is 15 mg ?

$$\begin{aligned}
\text{Child's dose} &= (15 \times 6) \div (6 + 12) \text{ mg} \\
&= 90 \div 18 \\
&= \tfrac{90}{18} = \tfrac{45}{9} = \tfrac{5}{1} \\
&= 5 \text{ mg}
\end{aligned}$$

Example 2: A girl of 8 years is to have atropine pre-operatively. If the adult dose is 0·6 mg, how much should she have?

$$\begin{aligned}
\text{Child's dose} &= (0{\cdot}6 \times 8) \div (8 + 12) \text{ mg} \\
&= 4{\cdot}8 \div 20 \\
&= \frac{\overset{24}{\cancel{48}}}{10} \times \frac{1}{\underset{10}{\cancel{20}}} = \frac{24}{100} \\
&= 0{\cdot}24 \text{ mg}
\end{aligned}$$

Fried's Rule is suitable for children under 12 months. The rule states that a suitable child's dose is calculated by multiplying the adult dose by the child's age *in months* and dividing by 150.

$$\text{Child's dose} = \frac{\text{Adult's dose} \times \text{age in months}}{150}$$

Example 1: How much of a drug can a child of 9 months have if the adult dose is 10 mg?

Child's dose $= 10 \times 9 \div 150$ mg

$$= \frac{\overset{2}{\cancel{10}} \times \overset{3}{9}}{\underset{\underset{5}{\underset{\cancel{10}}{\cancel{30}}}}{\cancel{150}}} = \frac{3}{5} = 0 \cdot 6 \text{ mg}$$

Example 2: The adult dose of syrup of senna is 6 ml. How much can be given to a child of 4 months?

Child's dose

$$= \frac{6 \times \overset{2}{\cancel{4}}}{\underset{\underset{25}{\cancel{50}}}{\cancel{150}}} = \frac{4}{25} = 0 \cdot 16 \text{ ml}$$

A further and more accurate method of stating dosage which is applicable to children and adults alike is to state the dose as so many milligrams, etc., per pound or kilogram of body weight. In order to find the correct dose it is necessary to weigh the patient, which is not always immediately practicable.

Example 1: Find the dose of streptomycin suitable for a child weighing 3 stone if the quantity to be given is 6 milligrams per pound.

Weight of child $= 3$ stone

$\qquad\qquad\quad = 3 \times 14$ pounds $= 42$ pounds

$\therefore$ Dose $= 42 \times 6$ mg

$\qquad\qquad = 252$ mg

$\qquad\qquad$ (roughly $\frac{1}{4}$ gramme)

Now consider this same problem using metric weights

throughout. The quantity of 6 mg per pound is multiplied by 2·2 to show the quantity given per kilogram

$$\therefore \text{dose} = 19\cdot09 \times (6 \times 2\cdot2) \text{ mg}$$
$$= 251\cdot988 \text{ mg}$$

(again approximately $\frac{1}{4}$ gramme)

Exercises

Calculate suitable doses from the following:

1. Child of 6 years.   Adult dose 1 ml nepenthe.
2. Child of 5 years.   Adult dose 100 mg phenytoin.
3. Child of 4 years.   Adult dose 0·6 mg atropine.
4. Child of 9 years.   Adult dose 500 mg sulphamethoxypyridazine.
5. Child of 10 years.   Adult dose dichloralphenazone 1·3 g.
6. Child of 3 months.   Adult dose 15 ml ephedrine hydrochloride mixture.
7. Child of 6 months.   Adult dose 300 mg syrup of ferrous gluconate.
8. How much Thiabendazole should be given to a patient weighing 44 kg if the dose is 25 mg per kg of body weight?

Now Try a Few Practical Problems Yourself

1. How would you give a patient an injection of Omnopon 15 mg from an ampoule marked 20 mg?
2. Prepare 2 pints of lotion strength 1 in 120 from a stock bottle of strength 1 in 20.
3. How much potassium permanganate solution 50% is required to prepare a general bath containing 90 litres of 2% strength?
4. Sodium hypochlorite 5% is supplied to the ward. How much will be required to make 2·5 litres 1 in 80 for babies' bottles?
5. How much silver nitrate solution strength 1 in 1000

must be used to prepare 1200 ml of solution strength 1 in 3000 for irrigation of the bladder? How much distilled water should be added?

6. An insulin bottle is marked 40 units per ml. How much will contain 25 units?

7. A bottle of morphine sulphate solution is labelled 15 mg in 2 ml. How much must be drawn up if it is required to give 10 mg?

8. An ampoule of solution is marked Pethidine Hyd 100 mg, Promethazine Hyd 50 mg in 2 ml. If 1·5 ml are injected how much pethidine and how much promethazine have been administered?

9. How much sudol 1 in 20 is required to make a quart of 1 in 160?

10. How would you prepare 600 ml of chlorhexidine of strength 1 in 1500 from a stock of 1 in 1000?

11. How much magnesium sulphate solution 1 in 5 is needed to make 300 ml of 1 in 20?

12. How much 1 in 2000 solution is needed to make 200 ml of 1 in 5000?

13. If 60 mg of morphine is dissolved in 4 ml of water, how much contains 20 mg?

14. Sodium citrate $2\frac{1}{2}\%$ is required as an anticoagulant for blood. How would you make 10 oz from 10% stock?

15. How much water must be added to 300 ml of 20% strength glucose to make it 5%?

16. Prepare 200 ml of Cetrimide 0·1% solution from stock of 1%.

17. How much 10% solution of povidine-iodine is required to make 250 ml of 1 in 25?

18. How much 20% alcohol solution can be made from 1 litre of 95%?

19. Prepare 1000 ml of 1 in 8000 potassium permanganate solution from 0·1% stock.

20. Make 250 ml cocaine solution 1% from 2%.

14
Thermometry

QUITE early in man's search for knowledge it was realized
that an accurate instrument for measuring temperature
changes was required. Answers to questions such as, 'How
much hotter or colder is this substance now that I have
experimented with it?' or 'Is today's temperature more or
less than yesterday's?' needed urgent answers in precise terms
before real advances could take place.

Much of the early work done on temperature was done by
men who were seeking to enhance their country's sea power.
It was beginning to be realized that wind strengths and changes
were connected with temperature in adjoining areas, and as
ships were dependent entirely on the winds, there would be
definite advantages to the navies that could predict how the
wind was going to blow, just as present-day meteorologists
supply the information on which our air fleets rely. Without
thermometers a serious gap is left.

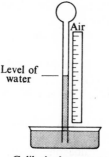

Galileo's thermometer

Galileo, the sixteenth-century genius, invented among all his other wonderful creations a kind of thermometer. This he did in 1593 and it is surprising that such a simple instrument was not invented before. It is something that any nurse could set up for herself. It consists of a flask with a cork in its neck through which passes a glass tube. This is turned upside down with the end of the tube under the surface of some water in a glass. The air in the glass bulb is heated thus causing it to expand and some of it will bubble away from the end of the tubing. When the air is allowed to cool some water is drawn up into the tubing. The level of the water in the tube will then rise and fall with even slight changes in room temperature. With an ordinary wall thermometer used as a guide it is possible to graduate the tubing quite accurately.

In spite of the extreme sensitivity of this thermometer it has certain drawbacks that make it unsuitable for general use. For one thing, it is bulky and easily broken; variations in atmospheric pressure will also cause the water to rise and fall in the tube independently of temperature; a very long tube indeed would be required for large temperature ranges. It was not long before better thermometers were invented.

Rey, a French doctor, in 1632, used a small bulb and tube filled with water with the end of the tube sealed, quite similar to our mercury filled thermometers, but larger. The water expanded along the tube when the bulb was warmed. He used to to detect rises in body temperature and to him can go the honour of inventing the first 'clinical thermometer'. This was quite useless to the climatologists, however. The water froze at low temperatures and between 4°C and 0°C showed an apparent rise in temperature owing to the peculiar property that water has of expanding instead of contracting between those temperatures.

The Florentine Academy took the next steps leading up to 'modern' thermometry. They established the principle that it was necessary to have two easily determined temperatures, one high and one low, that were constant. Any thermometer could then be graduated so that 10 degrees meant the same on one as it meant on any other. These two 'fixed points' would have to be the temperatures of easily available things and were chosen as the temperature of snow or ice during the severest frost of the winter and the rectal temperature of cows or deer. The space in between these two points was then divided into forty or eighty equal divisions or degrees. The winter temperatures of Florence must have been remarkably constant as several of these Florentine thermometers came to light recently and all showed the temperature of melting ice to be at $13\frac{1}{2}$ degrees. Nowadays we recognize that these temperatures are far too variable to be of practical use for the accuracy that we demand, but at that time the principle constituted a remarkable advance.

The second achievement was the substitution of alcohol for water as the expanding fluid. Alcohol was unfreezable at that time so that comparatively low temperatures could then be recorded. In addition, alcohol expands at a constant rate throughout the whole range of temperatures. Its greatest drawback was that it has a boiling point slightly lower than that of water and could not be used for higher temperatures.

Mercury was first used by a Parisian astronomer, Boulliau, in 1659, and there the matter stood for nearly 50 years until Fahrenheit invented his thermometer in 1712.

Fahrenheit took a small glass bulb with a narrow glass tube leading from it and filled the bulb with mercury. He then heated the mercury until it expanded to fill the tube completely. The end of the tube was then sealed in a flame, and as the mercury cooled it shrank back into the bulb leaving a vacuum behind it. This is the type of thermometer we are familiar with today. His next step was to establish two fixed points on the stem of the thermometer. For his lower fixed point he put his thermometer into a mixture of ammoniated salt and ice believing this to be the coldest temperature possible to attain. This was marked zero. His upper fixed point was obtained by placing the thermometer in boiling water. The level to which the mercury rose was marked on the stem and this was labelled 212 degrees. Why Fahrenheit chose these particular figures will forever remain a mystery. On this scale the temperature of melting ice is 32 degrees and, as this temperature is the one used to determine the lower fixed points in the two other major scales, it is of far more importance than Fahrenheit's zero. This should be remembered as it is of some importance when the question of conversion from one scale to another is to be considered.

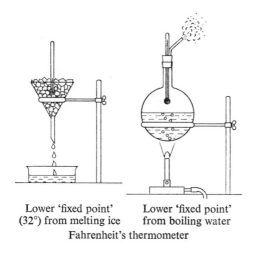

Lower 'fixed point'　　Lower 'fixed point'
(32°) from melting ice　　from boiling water
Fahrenheit's thermometer

In 1742, Celsius, a Swede working in Switzerland, introduced what has been known as the Centigrade scale. He used the temperatures of freezing and boiling water as his lower and upper fixed points. The distance between these two points he divided into 100 equal divisions or degrees. At first he called the upper one 0 degrees and the lower one 100 degrees but 9 years later these were reversed by a fellow worker and were named as we know them today with the freezing point of water at 0 degrees and the boiling point of water at 100 degrees.

The term Centigrade is used in some other countries to denote fractions of a right angle. Therefore when agreement was reached on the International System of Units it was decided that the name 'degree Centigrade' will be replaced by the name 'degree Celsius'.

Conversion from one Scale to Another

Because the Fahrenheit scale is still used extensively in Great Britain it is the scale that conveys most meaning to many nurses. When one hears that the temperature on a certain day was 90°F in the shade, a picture of oppressive heat is

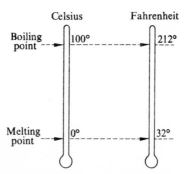

Equivalent point on the two scales

conjured up in one's mind. But if one hears that the temperature was 32·2°C in the shade, it conveys very little impression unless one has become used to dealing with the Celsius scale, and then one realizes that it is the same thing. It is a question of familiarity. Until such familiarity has been cultivated it is necessary to be able to convert from one scale to the other.

There are two methods for conversion, both of which we shall consider.

Method 1

The rules for conversion are very simple. Let us write them down and then examine them to see how they are derived.

(1) **To convert degrees Celsius to degrees Fahrenheit multiply the degrees Celsius by $\frac{9}{5}$ and then add 32.**

(2) **To convert degrees Fahrenheit to degrees Celsius, subtract 32 from the degrees Fahrenheit and then multiply by $\frac{5}{9}$.**

The usual difficulty that nurses encounter is to remember whether to multiply by $\frac{5}{9}$ or $\frac{9}{5}$. As this can be worked out from first principles in a few moments it need not constitute a major problem. Both scales use the same fixed points, the freezing and boiling points of water. Therefore 0°C and 32°F are equal. So too are 100°C and 212°F. Between 0 and 100 there are obviously 100 divisions, and between 32 and 212 there are 180 divisions. Hence 100 Celsius degrees covers the same range as 180 Fahrenheit degrees. If 100 Celsius divisions is equal to 180 Fahrenheit divisions, 1 Celsius degree must equal 180 divided by 100 Fahrenheit degrees. By simplification, $\frac{180}{100}$ becomes $\frac{9}{5}$. Why this should present any difficulty is hard to see. If a person were to say, 'Here are 100 counters made of black plastic. They have the same value as 180 red beads', anyone could answer the question 'How much is one black counter worth?' This leads logically to the answers to, 'How much are 10, 15 or 75 counters worth?'

The same applies to degrees. If $1°C = \frac{9}{5}°F$, $10°C = \frac{9}{5} \times 10°F$, $20°C = \frac{9}{5} \times 20°F$, $75°C = \frac{9}{5} \times 75°F$, and so on.

To each of these answers must be added 32. This is because the starting point of both scales is the freezing point of water which is called zero on the Celsius scale but is called 32 on the Fahrenheit scale. In other words, the Fahrenheit scale has got a 'start' on the Celsius, and its 'handicap' must be added after the multiplication if the comparison is going to be 'fair'.

Converting from Fahrenheit to Celsius is carried out

by reversing the process. The 'handicap' must be removed first of all so we start by subtracting 32. The next step is to multiply the remainder by $\frac{5}{9}$. This figure is derived in the following way. If 180 Fahrenheit degrees are equal to 100 Celsius degrees, one Fahrenheit degree equals 100 divided by 180 Celsius degrees. $\frac{100}{180} = \frac{5}{9}$ when the simplification has been completed. Hence, if 1 Fahrenheit degree equals $\frac{5}{9}$ of a Celsius degree, 10 Fahrenheit degrees equals $10 \times \frac{5}{9}$ Celsius degrees and so on.

Example 1: Convert 98·6°F to the Celsius scale.

(*a*)   Subtract 32

$$98·6 - 32 = 66·6$$

(*b*)   Multiply by $\frac{5}{9}$

$$\overset{7·4}{\cancel{66·6}} \times \frac{5}{\underset{1}{\cancel{9}}} = 7·4 \times \frac{5}{1}$$

$$= 37$$

Therefore *98·6°F = 37°C*

Example 2: Convert 59°F to the Celsius scale.

(*a*)   59 − 32 = 27

(*b*) $\overset{3}{\cancel{27}} \times \frac{5}{\underset{1}{\cancel{9}}} = 15$

Therefore *59°F = 15°C*

Example 3: Convert 12·2°F to the Celsius scale.

(*a*)   12·2 − 32 = minus 19·8

(*b*)   minus $\overset{2·2}{\cancel{19·8}} \times \frac{5}{\underset{1}{\cancel{9}}} =$ minus 11

Therefore *12·2°F = minus 11°C*

Now in the reverse direction:

Example 1: Convert 10°C to the Fahrenheit scale.

(*a*)   Multiply by $\frac{9}{5}$

$$\overset{2}{\cancel{10}} \times \frac{9}{\cancel{5}} = 18$$
$$\phantom{10 \times \frac{9}{5} = 18}_{1}$$

(*b*)   Add 32

$$18 + 32 = 50$$
Therefore *10°C = 50°F*

Example 2: Convert 95°C to the Fahrenheit scale.

$$(a) \quad \overset{19}{\cancel{95}} \times \frac{9}{\cancel{5}} = 171$$
$$\phantom{(a) \quad 95 \times \frac{9}{5} = 171}_{1}$$

$$(b) \quad 171 + 32 = 203$$
Therefore *95°C = 203°F*

Example 3: Convert minus 5°C to the Fahrenheit scale.

(*a*)   minus 5 × $\frac{9}{5}$ = minus 9
(*b*)   minus 9 + 32 = 23

Therefore *minus 5°C = 23°F*

Method 2

This method may be found by some people to be easier to remember than the first. The steps are as follows:

1st step.   add 40
2nd step.   (*a*)   multiply by $\frac{5}{9}$ to convert from the Fahrenheit scale to the Celsius scale.

or

(*b*)   multiply by $\frac{9}{5}$ to convert from the Celsius scale to the Fahrenheit scale

3rd step.   Now the 1st step is reversed, that is, 40 is deducted from the total

To allow this method to be compared with the first method let us try it on the problems already worked.

Example 1: Convert 98·6°F to the Celsius scale.

(*a*)   add 40

$$98·6 + 40 = 138·6$$

(*b*)   multiply by $\frac{5}{9}$

$$\frac{\overset{15·4}{\cancel{138·6} \times 5}}{\underset{1}{9}} = 77·0$$

(*c*)   subtract 40

$$77 - 40 = 37°C$$

Example 2: Convert 59°F to the Celsius scale.

(*a*)   add 40

$$59 + 40 = 99$$

(*b*)   multiply by $\frac{5}{9}$

$$\frac{\overset{11}{\cancel{99} \times 5}}{\underset{1}{9}} = 55$$

(*c*)   subtract 40

$$55 - 40 = 15°C$$

Example 3: Convert 12·2°F to the Celsius scale.

(*a*)   add 40

$$12·2 + 40 = 52·2$$

(*b*)   multiply by $\frac{5}{9}$

$$\frac{\overset{5·8}{\cancel{52·2} \times 5}}{\underset{1}{9}} = 29·0$$

(*c*)   subtract 40

$$29 - 40 = -11°C$$

Next we shall work in the reverse direction again.

Example 1: Convert 10°C to the Fahrenheit scale.

(*a*)   add 40

$$10 + 40 = 50$$

(*b*)   multiply by $\frac{9}{5}$

$$\frac{\overset{10}{\cancel{50}} \times 9}{\underset{1}{\cancel{5}}} = 90$$

(*c*)   subtract 40

$$90 - 40 = 50°F$$

Example 2: Convert 95°C to the Fahrenheit scale.

(*a*)   add 40

$$95 + 40 = 135$$

(*b*)   multiply by $\frac{9}{5}$

$$\frac{\overset{27}{\cancel{135}} \times 9}{\underset{1}{\cancel{5}}} = 243$$

(*c*)   subtract 40

$$243 - 40 = 203°F$$

Example 3: Convert minus 5°C to the Fahrenheit scale.

(*a*)   add 40

$$-5 + 40 = 35$$

(*b*)   multiply by $\frac{9}{5}$

$$\frac{\overset{7}{\cancel{35}} \times 9}{\underset{1}{\cancel{5}}} = 63$$

(*c*)   subtract 40

$$63 - 40 = 23°F$$

Exercises

1. Give four reasons why mercury is a better liquid to use in thermometers than water.

2. What disadvantages are there to water as a thermometer liquid? Are there any advantages?

3. Convert each of the following to the Fahrenheit scale:

(a) 3°C	(b) 18°C	(c) 25·5°C	(d) 100°C
(e) 36°C	(f) 42°C	(g) 50°C	(h) 70°C

4. Convert each of the following to the Celsius scale:

(a) 41°F	(b) 77°F	(c) 55·4°F	(d) 104°F
(e) 86°F	(f) 78·8°F	(g) 365·9°F	(h) 212°F

5. State which of the following are true and which false:

(a) 0°C = 0°F	(b) 32°F = 0°C
(c) 98·6°F = 37°C	(d) minus 40°C = minus 40°F
(e) 40°F = 40°C	(f) 100°F = 100°C
(g) 92°F = 60°C	

The Clinical Thermometer

It is possible to take a person's temperature with an ordinary thermometer, especially if it is used rectally, but it is not an easy matter. The glass is usually so thick that the thermometer has to be left in contact with the tissues for a considerable length of time. The bore of the tube is comparatively large compared with that of a clinical thermometer and consequently requires more heat to cause the mercury to expand. The heat lost from the stem of the thermometer may equal that gained from the body if the stem is very long, so the mercury will never be able to climb to a true reading. There is no provision made to prevent the mercury contracting back into the bulb when it is removed from the tissues so that it would have to be read in situ.

All these disadvantages have been overcome in the clinical

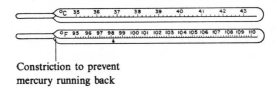

Constriction to prevent
mercury running back

A clinical thermometer

thermometer. As such thermometers will be used only to record temperatures at which living tissue exists, it would be pointless to make them so that they are capable of registering the freezing point or the boiling point of water. It is generally considered that animal tissues will die if they are kept at temperatures much below 35°C or over 43·3°C for more than a very short time. Hence a standard clinical thermometer need only register between these limits. Special thermometers are used for recording the sub-normal temperatures of some elderly people and of patients undergoing operations involving hypothermic techniques.

Secondly, to use glass as thick as that used in other types of thermometers is likely to cause considerable delay in the registering of the temperature. This is time that can be ill afforded in the running of a busy ward. Therefore the glass of clinical thermometers is quite thin particularly round the bulb.

Thirdly, there is need for great accuracy. Far more so than is the case with the temperature of a room or boiler where accuracy to one degree is quite sufficient. This accuracy can be attained by making the bore of the thermometer very fine so that the mercury travels further along the stem as it expands. This allows for graduations of one-fifth of a degree or less.

Fourthly, the mercury having expanded, it must be prevented from returning into the bulb as it cools after removal from the body. This is achieved by making the bore of the stem even smaller at a point just above the bulb. Obviously it must not be made so narrow that the mercury cannot be forced back into the bulb, and every nurse soon learns the knack of 'shaking down' the thermometer with a flick of the wrist. Some thermometers are easier to 'shake down' than others, indicating that the size of the constriction varies from one thermometer to another.

Many clinical thermometers have a triangular cross section so that the mercury may be seen more easily. The effect of this peculiar cross section is to magnify the fine hair-like thread of mercury. Sometimes the glass behind the thread of mercury is coloured, usually white, but sometimes red or blue. The silvery colour stands out more clearly than if the glass behind were transparent.

Most clinical thermometers have the time that it takes to record engraved into the glass at the back. Some are 3-min thermometers, some 2-min, some 1- or $\frac{1}{2}$- or even $\frac{1}{4}$-min. If a 3-min one is compared with a $\frac{1}{2}$-minute one, it becomes obvious immediately that much of the thickness of the glass has been sacrificed for the sake of speed of recording. You can have a comparatively strong one that takes a much longer time to record or you can have a fragile one that records quickly. Even so, many nurses find that the time recorded on the back is quite unreliable even with an expensive thermometer, and usually they prefer to take no chances and keep the thermometer in position for a full 3 min in spite of what is stated on the back.

Conversion Tables for Transposing Fahrenheit and Celsius

To use the table for conversion from Celsius to Fahrenheit split the temperature into tens, units and decimals and look up the figures for each. Write these down under each other and then add them to find the temperature in degrees Fahrenheit. For example, to convert 48·6°C look up the figures for 40°, then 8° and lastly 0·6°. Enter them thus

$$
\begin{array}{r}
104 \\
14\cdot4 \\
1\cdot08 \\
\hline
119\cdot48
\end{array}
$$

Therefore 48·6°C = 119·48°F

The table can be used for temperatures higher than 109·9°C but, as the first column of Fahrenheit degrees has already had 32 added to make up for the difference between the zero points in the two scales, care must be taken to subtract 32 when looking up the converted figure for the 'tens'. For instance, to find the equivalent of 160°C look up the figure for 100°, then the figure for 60°. Now 32 has been added to both of these figures already, so one lot of 32 must be taken off again to give the final figure. Hence, 100°C = 212°F, 60°C = 140°F and 160° C= 212 + 140 − 32 = 320°F.

Table to convert Celsius to Fahrenheit

°C	°F	°C	°F	°C	°F
0	32	1	1·8	0·1	0·18
10	50	2	3·6	0·2	0·36
20	68	3	5·4	0·3	0·54
30	86	4	7·2	0·4	0·72
40	104	5	9·0	0·5	0·9
50	122	6	10·8	0·6	1·08
60	140	7	12·6	0·7	1·26
70	158	8	14·4	0·8	1·44
80	176	9	16·2	0·9	1·62
90	194				
100	212				

The second table is for conversion from Fahrenheit to Celsius and is used in the same way. Here again temperatures higher than 219·9°F can be converted with a similar proviso and that is that the amount of 17·8 must be added to the figure found for anything in the 'tens'. For example 280°F is first split into 200 and 80. 200°F = 93·3°C, 80°F = 26·7°C, therefore 280°F = 93·3 + 26·7 + 17·8 = 137·8°C.

Table to convert Fahrenheit to Celsius

°F	°C	°F	°C	°F	°C
30	− 1·1	1	0·56	0·1	0·06
40	4·4	2	1·11	0·2	0·11
50	10·0	3	1·67	0·3	0·17
60	15·6	4	2·22	0·4	0·22
70	21·1	5	2·78	0·5	0·28
80	26·7	6	3·33	0·6	0·33
90	32·2	7	3·89	0·7	0·39
100	37·8	8	4·44	0·8	0·44
110	43·3	9	5·0	0·9	0·5
120	48·9				
130	54·4				
140	60·0				
150	65·6				
160	71·1				
170	76·7				
180	82·2				
190	87·8				
200	93·3				
210	98·9				

15
Heat and Calories

TEMPERATURE is a measurement that tells us the degree of hotness of a substance. It tells us whether something is hotter or cooler than another object without giving us the slightest indication as to how much **heat** that particular object contains. A good analogy can be made between the quality of wetness in liquids. We can say that rain water is wetter than sea water, or that normal saline is wetter than Epsom salts solution, just as we can say that such and such an object is hotter than another. To say that one liquid is wetter than another gives us no clue to the quantity of water just as the temperature gives us no clue to the amount of heat.

It is possible to have a kettle of water containing 1 litre and another containing 4 litres, both have exactly the same temperature, but there will be four times as much **heat** in the 4 litres as there is in the 1 litre. Putting this another way round makes it self-evident. In order to boil both these kettles it will take four times as long to boil the 4 litre one as it will to boil the other, provided the size of the gas jet remains the same for both. In other words, one has to put four times as much heat into the large quantity as into the small quantity.

One can think of many examples to illustrate this point. For instance, which would you rather take to bed on a cold night, a hot water bottle with a 2 litre capacity or a baby's hot water bottle containing $\frac{1}{4}$ of a litre? Why? Because the larger one stays hot longer of course. It contains more heat than the smaller one and it takes longer for the heat to dissipate. Or again, if you had to iron sheets with an old-fashioned flat iron, would you choose a large one or a small one? A large one because, even though they are heated to

the same temperature in the first place, the large one will
absorb more heat and will stay hot longer in consequence.

A simple experiment can be performed to show that
different quantities of water at the same temperature contain
different quantities of heat in proportion to their volume.
Take a beaker of water containing 50 ml and stand a test

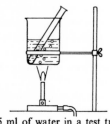

5 ml of water in a test tube
standing in
50 ml of boiling water

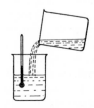

50 ml of boiling water
added to
50 ml of cold water

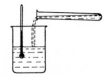

5 ml of boiling water
added to
50 ml of cold water

tube in it containing 5 ml. Heat the beaker over a jet. Take
the temperature of the water in the beaker and that in the test
tube. They should be the same. Now put two more beakers
of the same size each containing 50 ml of tap water. Take
the temperature of this water. Into one pour the water from
the heated beaker and into the other pour the water from the
test tube. Now take the temperatures of the mixtures. What
is the **increase** in temperature in each case? It will be seen
that the larger quantity of hot water has increased the temperature of the cold water by ten times the amount achieved by

the small quantity, which indicates that the larger quantity contained ten times as much heat as the smaller quantity even though they were heated to the same temperature.

Units of Heat

Now that it is clear that temperature is not the same as quantity of heat it can be seen that it has been necessary to invent units that will measure quantities of heat. As in all other cases of measurement a unit or standard is required for purposes of comparison.

The unit quantity of heat is called **a calorie** and is defined **as the quantity of heat that will raise the temperature of one gramme of water by one degree Celsius.**

The quantity of heat required to raise the temperature of 2 g of water by 1°C is therefore 2 calories. Similarly if 6 g of water is heated sufficient to raise its temperature by 1°C it will have taken up 6 calories. If 10 g are raised 12°C it will have received $10 \times 12 = 120$ calories, the number of calories being equal to the weight of water in grammes multiplied by the rise in temperature in degrees Celsius.

There is also a unit in the British measurements called a British Thermal Unit or B.T.U. for short. This is defined as the amount of heat required to raise the temperature of 1 lb of water through 1°F. This is equivalent to 252 calories. Calories and British Thermal Units are rather small quantities when it comes to measuring the heat value of gas supplies or food substances and for these purposes larger units have been devised. Dietetic Calories are equivalent to 1000 of the calories that are written about here. We shall come across dietetic Calories later in this book. The heating power of gas is measured in therms, one of which is equivalent to 100,000 B.T.U. How the supply of gas can be adjusted to the demand for it may be illustrated by an example. An iron kettle weighs 3 lb and the water in it weighs 5 lb. Taking the specific heat of iron as $\frac{1}{9}$, the 3 lb kettle is equivalent to $3 \times \frac{1}{9}$ lb of water which equals $\frac{1}{3}$ lb. Hence the weight of the kettle plus the

water is equivalent of $5\frac{1}{3}$ lb of water. Therefore it will take
$5\frac{1}{3}$ B.T.U. to raise its temperature through 1°F, and to raise
the temperature from room temperature, say 62°F, to boiling
(212°F), i.e. through 150°F, it will take $5\frac{1}{3} \times 150 = 800$
B.T.U. If we know that the heating power of 1 cubic foot of
gas is 400 B.T.U. it is obvious that it will take 2 cubic feet
to boil the kettle. In similar fashion it can be discovered how
much gas it will take to boil any quantity of water in any size
boiler and if the gas is priced at so much per cubic foot, an
approximate estimate of keeping the boiler going can be made.

Specific Heat

Mention was made in the foregoing illustration of the
'specific heat' of iron. This needs explanation. It has been said
that it takes 1 calorie to raise the temperature of 1 g *of water*
through 1°C. It is found upon experiment that no other
substance (with the exception of hydrogen under constant
pressure) needs quite so much heat to raise its temperature.
In other words, substances other than water get hot more
quickly than water when subjected to the same heating source.
They also cool more quickly when that heating source is
removed. The amount of heat that 1 g of a substance needs
to raise its temperature 1°C is called its specific heat.

The word specific is a familiar one to nurses. For instance,
some diseases are best treated by a drug that has a specific
effect on that disease such as salicylic acid in acute rheuma-
tism, or streptomycin on tuberculosis. Yet again, certain
diseases cause certain signs and symptoms that are specific
for that disease and occur in no other, like Corrigan's pulse
in aortic stenosis. Or still further, that antibodies in the blood
stream are specific for certain toxins and have no effect on
the toxins of other organisms. So too with the specific heats
of substances. Each substance needs a certain amount of heat
to raise the temperature of 1 g through 1°C.

Water, by definition, needs 1 calorie for this. Hence its
specific heat is 1. If we do some experiments and find that the

temperature of 1 g of iron filings is raised by 1°C after supplying it with only 0·125 calories we can say the specific heat of iron is 0·125. The practical application of this is that we can predict the rise in temperature that will result from supplying any weight of any substance with a certain quantity of heat by multiplying the weight by the specific heat and dividing this product into the number of calories supplied.

Looking at a list of some specific heats interesting facts emerge.

Sand	0·19	Water	1·00
Turpentine	0·42	Steel	0·126
Aluminium	0·21	Zinc	0·096
Cast Iron	0·125	Copper	0·097
Mercury	0·03	Tin	0·056

The specific heat of sand is 0·19 while that of water is 1. This means that land, particularly land bare of vegetation, will get much hotter than the adjoining water under the action of the sun. It will get five times hotter approximately or rather, it will get hot five times as quickly. At night it will lose its heat five times faster than the water. Hence the relative coolness of sea breezes during the later part of the day, and the relative warmth of the same breezes in the later part of the night.

Aluminium has a higher specific gravity than cast iron, so that if saucepans of these two metals having the same weight are used to boil water, the water in the cast iron one will boil first. In actual practice however, it is found that aluminium, being so much less dense than cast iron, is more suitable as the saucepans can be made of much thinner metal.

The specific heat of mercury is very low; only 0·03. This means that mercury will absorb heat about thirty-three times faster than water and a simple experiment can be performed to show that this is so.

Take two beakers of the same size and place in one 100 g of water. Place in the other 100 g of mercury. Take the temperatures of both liquids and note them. Place the beakers over bunsen flames of equal size and intensity to ensure as near as possible that both liquids are receiving heat at the same rate. Heat for 3 minutes. Take the temperatures of both liquids at the end of this time. Subtract the starting temperatures from the final temperatures to find the rise in both cases and it will be apparent that the mercury has gained approximately thirty-three times as much heat as the water.

From this emerges a very good reason for using mercury instead of water in clinical thermometers. If such a thermometer were filled with water it would take more than half an hour for it to register where the mercury thermometer takes only 1 minute.

Another glance at the list of specific heats reveals that zinc and copper have lower specific heats than steel. This explains why they are often used for making sterilizers. Tin would be even better if it were not for the fact that it melts at a temperature of only 232°C.

Latent Heat

Although it takes 1 calorie to raise the temperature of 1 g of water 1°C, there comes a time when the temperature of the water will rise no further no matter how many more calories are supplied. This point is reached when the water starts to boil and from then on it will stay at a temperature of 100°C while it gradually 'boils away'. In other words, the calories are still being absorbed but they fail to raise the temperature. Instead they provide the energy for the water to change into steam. The number of calories required to change 1 g of a liquid substance into a gas is called the latent heat of that particular substance. To be more accurate, it is called the latent heat of vaporization of that particular substance and this distinguishes it from the amount of heat required to change a solid to a liquid which is referred to as the latent heat of fusion of the solid. Considerably more calories are required to bring about these changes of state, and an experiment can be done to find out how much is required to change water into steam.

Place 5 g (5 ml) of water in a beaker and take its temperature. Place the beaker over a flame and note carefully how long it takes the water to boil. It will then be at 100°C so there is no need to take the temperature again. Subtract the original temperature from 100 to find the rise in temperature, and this figure multiplied by 5, the weight of the water, will show how many calories have been absorbed all together. This last figure divided by the time that it took the water to boil will indicate fairly accurately the rate at which the flame is delivering heat. Continue to boil the water with an undiminished flame and note exactly how long it takes to 'boil dry', i.e. how long it takes for the 5 g of water to be evaporated completely into steam. The rate at which heat is being delivered has been discovered so, by multiplying the last time taken by the rate, the total number of calories required to evaporate 5 g of water is determined. Dividing this figure by 5 will tell us how many calories are required to evaporate 1 g and this is the latent heat of vaporization of water.

The completed calculations should look like this:

Weight of water	= 5 g
Initial temperature of the water	= 20°C
Final temperature of the water	= 100°C
Therefore the increase in temperature	= 80°C
Therefore the total number of calories delivered	= 80 × 5 calories
	= 400 calories
Time taken to boil the water	= 2 minutes
Therefore the flame delivers 400 ÷ 2 calories per minute	= 200 calories per minute
Time taken to evaporate all the water	= 14 minutes

Therefore the total heat used to
  vaporize 5 g of water $= 200 \times 14$ calories

The heat required to vaporize 1 g
  of water $= \dfrac{200 \times 14}{5}$ calories

$$= 40 \times 14$$
$$= 560$$

Therefore the latent heat of vaporization of water = 560 by this experiment.

Actually there will be some loss of heat to the beaker and the surrounding air which has not been accounted for, so the real figure is slightly lower at 536. Even so it proves a remarkable point, i.e. that substances need a considerable amount of energy in order to change their state from solid to liquid and from liquid to gas. This extra energy remains locked up in the molecules of the substance until a change takes place back into its original state whereupon all this energy is released again.

The latent heat of fusion of ice is 80. In other words, ice needs 80 calories per gramme to turn it into water. It also means that when water turns into ice it **releases** 80 calories per gramme. This principle has been used for heating purposes. It is possible to decompress water suddenly so that it turns into ice. The heat liberated from this process is then collected and used for heating air to circulate round buildings.

The very great latent heat of steam explains why a scald with steam is so much worse than one with boiling water. Every gramme of steam that condenses to water in contact with the skin liberates 536 calories while that amount of heat would be liberated by 50 g of hot water while cooling through 10 degrees.

Water evaporating imperceptibly from the skin takes 536 calories per gramme just the same as if it were boiling so that nature's mechanism for cooling the blood is a most efficient one.

Exercises

1. If an electric sterilizer containing 6 litres of water takes 20 min to boil from an original temperature of 20°C, how long is it safe to leave it before it boils dry? (Take the latent heat of steam to be 540.)

2. How often should a steam kettle containing 2 litres be refilled if it takes 1 hour for it to boil tap water at a temperature of 15°C?

Dietetic Calories

The normal calorie is far too small a quantity of heat to be of practical value in the study of dietetics, so a more manageable quantity has been devised. This is the 'Large' Calorie and it is the equivalent of 1000 ordinary calories. The dietetic Calorie should always be spelt with a capital 'C' to distinguish it from the small one, but this is often ignored in practice as the large calorie is the only one used in dietetics and confusion cannot arise provided newcomers to dietetics realize what they are dealing with from the start.

A dietetic Calorie can be defined as the amount of heat needed to raise the temperature of 1 litre of water through 1°C. In the English system it is the amount of heat needed to raise the temperature of 1 lb of water 4°F.

At first glance this seems to have little connection with the metabolism of carbohydrates and fats, but as both these substances are burnt in the body it is convenient to use heat units to measure their usefulness. The process of burning in the body is not greatly different from the burning of carbon compounds outside the body; wax candles, coal, petrol, gas, wood and paraffin are all carbon compounds that utilize oxygen to produce heat energy. Waste products result from the combustion, carbon dioxide and water, and these escape into the air. Inside the body carbohydrates, fats and proteins also utilize oxygen to produce energy with the production of the waste products carbon dioxide and water.

If a controlled experiment takes place, it is found that the oxygen needed to burn a certain amount of carbohydrate outside the body is almost constant, also the amount of carbon dioxide is constant. It is very likely therefore, that the same definite quantity of oxygen is needed to burn the same amount of carbohydrate inside the body, and the same amount of carbon dioxide is produced. Oxygen intake and carbon dioxide output can be measured readily and it is indeed found that dietary intake, oxygen intake and carbon dioxide output balance perfectly just as they do outside the body. In the case of carbohydrates catabolism is almost 100%, of fats it is about 95%, and of proteins about 92%, the unburnt portions of the fats and proteins escaping from the body as urea, creatine, uric acid, etc.

The amount of energy being produced inside the body cannot be measured directly, but as long as oxygen intake and carbon dioxide output remain constant factors, it is possible to work out mathematically the energy production. Most of the knowledge that we have regarding dietary requirements has been discovered in this way.

Basal Metabolic Rate

Certain body functions such as heart beat, respiration, maintenance of body temperature, circulation of blood and glandular secretion continue incessantly. These functions represent the absolute minimum activity that is necessary to keep a person alive and the rate at which substances are burnt to maintain these essential functions is termed the basal metabolic rate.

In order to measure this rate, the subject must be at absolute rest and digestion must have ceased. The usual time to take the measurements is first thing in the morning after fasting for at least 12 hr. A spirometer moves up and down as the subject breathes in and out of it, and these movements are recorded on a revolving drum. As the oxygen is used up a curve results, from which the amount of oxygen used is calculated. Carbon dioxide is absorbed into a suitable chemical which is weighed before and after the experiment, the difference in weight representing the amount of carbon dioxide exhaled. The basal metabolic rate is based on the respiratory quotient which is the figure resulting from dividing the amount of carbon dioxide by the amount of oxygen. If combustion in the body were complete the amount of carbon dioxide produced would be exactly equal to the amount of oxygen taken in and the respiratory quotient would be 1. As proteins and fats are not burned to completion, there is less carbon dioxide exhaled than there is oxygen inhaled so that the respiratory quotient in normal healthy individuals is about 0·85. This represents a Calorie requirement of roughly 1500 for a person of average height and weight, say 5 ft 8 in (172·5 cm), and 10 stone (63·4 kg).

In other wards, the average adult male requires food that will provide him with 1500 Calories merely to remain alive. Anything less in the diet means that he will start using stored glycogen; when that is exhausted, and the maximum amount that can be stored is about 540 g, the body fats are used, and last of all the tissue proteins. To do any sort of work, even the lightest imaginable, will require food intake over and above that needed to maintain basic metabolism.

The Calorie values of all the foodstuffs in general use have been worked out. A useful list will be found at the end of this chapter. One of the important tasks a nurse has to perform is to work out attractive menus from such lists having regard to the patient's illness and needs. This is a fascinating process as the paper work is going to be translated into actual plates of food and cups of liquid by the cooks, and if a nurse knows her patient really well, she can make the task even more enjoyable and mentally stimulating by including all the things that she knows are liked the most, or by substituting other foods when her patient's condition forbids certain things.

Calorie values per 100 grammes edible portion

Potato (fresh)	85	Lean beef	194
Wholemeal bread	262	Cheese	398
Sugar	387	Butter	716
Tinned pears	75	Cream	336
Cooked rice	100	Whole milk (per 100 ml)	65

Exercises

1. The following is for a patient's lunch:

Lean beef	60 g	Tinned pears	60 g
Potato	140 g	Cream	15 g
Butter	15 g		

Calculate the Calorie value from the list above.

2. A rice pudding containing the following items is enough for twelve people:

rice 120 g, sugar 120 g, milk 1·6 litre

What is the total Calorie value? What is the Calorie value of one portion?

3. What is the Calorie value of a cup of tea containing 120 ml water, 30 ml milk, and 10 g sugar?

4. A sweet for ten persons contains stewed fruit, sugar and cream with total Calorie values of 280, 250 and 250 respectively. What is the Calorie value per portion?

5. Which has the lower Calorie value, 60 g wholemeal bread plus 30 g cheese, or 280 ml of milk?

16
Pressure and its effects

ANYTHING resting on a surface exerts a downward force distributed over the resting surface equal to its own weight. A cube of metal weighing 1 kg and surfaces of 10 sq. cm on each side, exerts a force of 1 kg over 10 sq. cm. This is a **pressure** of (1000 ÷ 10) g on each sq. cm, i.e. 100 g per sq. cm. Pressure can be defined as force per unit area. This example is perfectly straightforward because the solid metal is tangible and solid. It can be weighed easily and the area of its regular sides can be determined easily. When calculating the pressure in liquids the density and depth of the liquid must be known. As liquids are practically incompressible the pressure will increase at a regular rate with the depth. This is expressed technically by saying that the pressure varies directly with the depth.

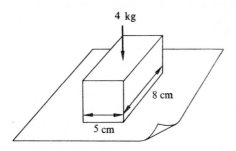

4 kg distributed over an area of 40 cm² = 100 g/cm²

With gases, however, there are several complicating factors. For one thing, the weight of a gas is not a constant factor. Since gas is compressible a given weight of gas can be made to occupy any desired volume. For instance, a gas cylinder may

have an internal volume of 60 litres; into this space it is possible to force 9·36 kg of air so that the air under those circumstances is weighing 156 g per litre. If this air is released
in an ordinary room it will expand to occupy something like
7200 cubic decimetres so that it now weighs approximately
1·3 g per cubic decimetre (litre). The empty cylinder still contains 60 litres of air with a weight of 78 g. If threequarters of
this air is sucked out with a suction pump, the remaining
quarter will then expand to fill the available space and its weight
will now be 0·325 g per litre. Furthermore the volume and
hence the weight of a gas will remain constant only if the temperature remains constant. The volume will increase by $\frac{1}{273}$ for
every rise of temperature of 1°C. These difficulties make it
impossible to perform accurate and reliable experiments unless
complicated equipment is available. Even so, nurses can perform
experiments that prove that air has *some* weight, which will
prove that it exerts pressure.

Take two compressed air cylinders (oxygen cylinders will do,
since the experiment is to prove that gas has weight), one full
and unused, the other empty. They should both be the same
size. Weigh them and compare the weights. The empty one
should weigh much less.

A second experiment can be done this way. Take a large
flask fitted with a rubber bung. Place some water in the flask
and weigh all together. Remove the bung and boil the water
vigorously for a few seconds. The steam from the water will
drive out all the air. Remove the flask from the heat and in
the same moment replace the bung, thus preventing air-re-
entering the flask. Let the flask cool thoroughly and weigh
again. It will be found that there is a slight loss of weight.
As air only weighs 1·3 g per litre under atmospheric pressure
and at a temperature of 0°C, the larger the flask used for
this experiment the more reliable the results will be.

Having determined that air has weight it must follow that
it exerts pressure. Indeed, when one considers that there is
an envelope of air around us that is many miles thick, it is

not surprising to find that it exerts a pressure of 15 lb to the square inch at sea level (approximately 1 kg per square centimetre). The pressure diminishes as one ascends through the atmosphere, as one would expect. The less air there is above one the less pressure it can exert.

The barometer is the instrument used for measuring air pressure. It is fairly easy to construct one as it consists of a glass tube about a yard long sealed at one end. This is filled with mercury and inverted into a bowl of mercury. The pressure of the air on the surface of the mercury in the bowl is sufficient to support only about 760 mm of the mercury; at

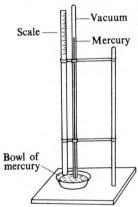

Simple mercury barometer

this point the tendency of the air to push mercury up the tube exactly counterbalances the tendency of the mercury to flow out of the tube. As the tube was originally filled and is about 92 cm long, when the tube is inverted some of the mercury will run out leaving a vacuum behind.

If it is desired to find out how long a tube must be to form a water barometer, it can be done mathematically quite easily. The density of mercury is 13·6 grammes per cubic centimetre, and atmospheric pressure is 760 mm (76 cm) of

mercury. The density of water is 1 gramme per cubic centimetre. Therefore it follows that if water is to be used the
column would need to be

$$76 \times 13 \cdot 6 = 1033 \cdot 6 \text{ cm}$$

Thus a water barometer tube would have to be at least 10·3 m
in length ($= 33 \cdot 8$ ft). Using English measurements the calculation can be made as follows: A cubic foot of water weighs
65 lb. Hence $\frac{15}{65}$ (15 divided by 65) cu. ft weighs 15 lb, so that
$\frac{15}{65}$ cu. ft will exert a downward force of 15 lb, and if it is contained in a tube with a cross section of 1 sq. in. none of the
water will flow out when the open end is inverted into a bowl of
water. Now volume is the product of length and area and, as
we stipulated that the area was to be 1 sq. in., the length must
be the volume divided by 1 sq. in. But the volume is $\frac{15}{65}$ cu. ft
so the length of the tube must be $\frac{15}{65}$ divided by 1 sq. in. These
must be in the same units before anything sensible emerges,
so convert the 1 sq. in. to square feet by dividing it by 144.

$$\text{Volume} = \tfrac{15}{65} \text{ cu. ft}$$
$$\text{Area} = \tfrac{1}{144} \text{ sq. ft}$$
$$\therefore \text{Length} = \tfrac{15}{65} \div \tfrac{1}{144} \text{ ft}$$
$$= \frac{15 \times 144}{65} \text{ ft}$$
$$= \frac{3 \times 144}{13} \text{ ft}$$
$$= 33\tfrac{1}{4} \text{ ft}$$

$$\begin{array}{r} 144 \\ 3 \\ \hline 13)\overline{432} \\ \hline 33\tfrac{1}{4} \text{ approx.} \end{array}$$

Therefore, a water barometer would have to be at least
34 ft long.

If the tube of a mercury barometer is fixed in an upright
position and a scale fitted alongside, observations can be
made over a period to see what variations occur in the height
of the mercury. It will be seen that the height is sometimes
more than 760 mm and sometimes less, which indicates that
the air pressure varies. The explanation for this lies in the fact
that air is a mixture of gases and one of these, water vapour,
varies in quantity at different times. As water vapour is lighter

than dry air when both are at the same temperature and pressure, it follows that a given volume of the air will be lighter the more water vapour it contains. Generally speaking, a fall in barometric pressure indicates a moister atmosphere and one can expect rain. This is not so all over the world, but it is usually the case in England.

Temperature also affects barometric pressure. Air expands as it gets warmer and a given volume will be lighter in consequence. Warm air is capable of containing more water vapour, which will depress the barometer still further.

The Effect of Pressure on Boiling Point

Under normal atmospheric pressure water boils at a temperature of 100°C (212°F). Steam issuing from such water is also at a temperature of 100°C (212°F) and is said to be moist or saturated steam. If the pressure is increased, as in a boiler, the boiling point of the water rises. With a pressure of 760 mm × 2 (15 lb above atmospheric pressure = 2 atmospheres) water boils at 121°C (250°F). At 760 mm × 3 (30 lb pressure above atmospheric pressure = 3 atmospheres) the boiling point is 133°C (271·4°F). The steam coming from such water is superheated, or dry steam, and is much used in hospitals and laboratories for sterilization purposes. All ordinary bacteria are killed in seconds by a temperature of 100°C (212°F) but spores may survive, after as much as twenty minutes exposure. They are killed by temperatures over 110°C (230°F) and heating in an autoclave is very suitable treatment. A further advantage is that superheated steam will not damage fabrics or cause scorching.

If increasing the pressure raises the boiling point it is reasonable to expect that the reverse is true, as indeed it is. An easy way to reduce the pressure on some water is to boil some in a flask. When it is boiling vigorously the steam will drive out all the air. If the flask is then corked quickly, taking care to remove the source of heat immediately, no air can get in and the water in the flask is no longer subjected to air

pressure. If the flask is then held under the cold water tap
the contained water will be seen to boil vigorously.

Another way of proving that reduced air pressure lowers
the boiling point is to take the temperature of water boiling
on the top of a mountain. Attempting to make tea with this
boiling water gives quite dramatic proof that it is not as hot
as water boiling at the foot of the mountain. This explains
perhaps why experienced mountaineers take a pressure cooker
as an essential part of equipment.

Safety Valves

The strength of a boiler is the strength of the weakest part
of its walls, just as the strength of a chain is the strength of its
weakest link. The difficulty with a boiler is to find its weak
spots and strengthen them. This is overcome by making the
boiler quite a lot stronger than is necessary for the job it
has to do and then making a 'weak spot' deliberately. This
artificial 'weak spot' is the safety valve. It consists of a metal
plug fitting closely into a hole in the top of the boiler. The
plug has a definite weight and a definite surface area inside
of which the pressure of the boiler can exert its force. When
the pressure reaches a certain point it overcomes the weight
of the plug and pushes it out. Some steam is released and the
pressure drops to within the safety margin and the plug falls
back into place.

Example 1: A boiler is constructed to produce steam at a
pressure of 50 lb per sq. in. above atmospheric pressure.
The safety valve has an internal surface area of $\frac{1}{2}$ sq. in. What
must its weight be?

$$\text{Steam pressure} = 50 \text{ lb per sq. in.}$$
$$\text{Area of safety valve} = \tfrac{1}{2} \text{ sq. in.}$$
$$\text{Therefore force needed to lift it} = 50 \times \tfrac{1}{2} \text{ lb}$$
$$= 25 \text{ lb}$$

Hence the weight of the safety valve is 25 lb.

Example 2: Another boiler is constructed to produce steam

at a pressure of 3·25 kg per square centimetre above atmospheric pressure. The safety valve has an internal surface area of 2 square centimetres. What must its weight be?

Steam pressure = 3·25 kg/sq. cm

Area of safety valve = 2 sq. cm

Therefore force needed to lift it = 3·25 × 2

= 6·5 kg

Thus the weight of the safety valve is 6·5 kg.

The Sphygmomanometer

This is an apparatus for recording blood pressure. It consists of a rubber 'cuff' which can be inflated by means of a rubber bulb-pump connected to the cuff by tubing. A further tube communicates with a mercury pressure gauge or manometer. The cuff is strapped round the patient's arm and sufficient air is pumped into it to compress the blood vessels in the arm. The air is then released, allowing the pressure to fall until the pulse just becomes apparent. The height of the mercury is then noted and this indicates the systolic pressure. This figure is usually expressed in millimetres and sometimes only the figures are written down, thus: 120 or 130.

Often the blood pressure is expressed as a fraction, e.g. 120/80 or 135/86 mmHg (Hg is the chemical symbol for mercury). The top figure is the systolic pressure. The lower figure is called the diastolic pressure and is the pressure existing in the heart and large arteries while the heart is resting between beats. This pressure is not so easy to determine as the systolic pressure and a stethoscope is required. When the diastolic pressure is to be taken, the systolic pressure is taken first, the stethoscope being applied to the bend of the elbow in order to hear when the heart beat recommences. The air pressure is then further reduced until the sound of the heart beat ceases to be heard. The manometer will be registering the diastolic pressure when the sound can still just be heard.

The Syringe

One of the commonest instruments depending on air pressure is the syringe. The piston must fit the barrel very closely or the syringe is inefficient. One explains the action of the syringe by saying that when the piston is withdrawn

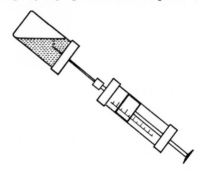

Inject a little air before drawing up

liquid is 'sucked up' into the barrel. It is more correct to say that when the piston is withdrawn liquid is pushed into the barrel by the pressure of the air on the surface of the liquid outside the syringe. Drawing back the piston reduces pressure inside the syringe while it remains constant outside, and liquids always flow from the high pressure region towards the low.

When a needle is inserted into a vein it is not unusual for the blood to force back the piston of the syringe without the operator having to exert any force himself. This indicates that the blood in that particular vein is under greater pressure than atmospheric.

Yet again, when extracting liquids from bottles with rubber caps on them it often happens that it becomes difficult to fill the syringe properly. The liquid inside such bottles is not open to the atmosphere, and as one extracts more and more liquid from them the contents remaining are subjected to lower and lower pressure. The point is soon reached where it is impossible to reduce the pressure in the syringe below that in the bottle and the liquid will not flow. This is easily overcome by injecting some air into the bottle beforehand, thus causing a pressure higher than atmospheric. The liquid will then flow into the syringe just as it does from a vein.

The Siphon

The easiest way to empty a sterilizer when it is not supplied with a tap is to siphon the water out. To do this, take a length of wide bore rubber tubing and fill it with water. Place one end of the tubing below the surface of the water in the sterilizer and the other end in a bucket. The water will then flow into the bucket provided the surface of the water in the bucket is below that in the sterilizer, and provided the end in the sterilizer stays under water.

Looking at this set-up it will be observed that the water must flow uphill through some part of the tubing, and this needs an explanation.

Air is pressing equally on the surface of the water in the sterilizer and on that in the bucket. In both cases there is a tendency for this air pressure to force water up the tube. This tendency is reduced by the water already in the tube tending to flow back into the sterilizer on the one hand and into the bucket on the other. If the tube leading to the bucket is longer than the part leading to the sterilizer the water it contains reduces the effectiveness of the air pressure by a greater amount on the bucket side. The effective air pressure is therefore greater on the surface of the water in the sterilizer and the water flows into the bucket. If we then raise the bucket from the floor so that it is higher than the sterilizer, we reverse the position and the water will flow from the bucket back into the sterilizer.

The commonest use of the siphon principle in everyday life is the lavatory flush. The pipe leading from the cistern to the pan is empty until the chain is pulled. The act of pulling the chain fills the pipe and as its end is below the water in the

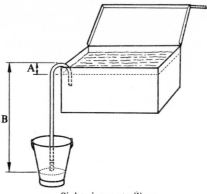

Siphoning a sterilizer

*The tendency of the water to flow into the bucket along ' B '
exceeds the tendency of the water to flow back into the
sterilizer along ' A '*

cistern, water flows down to flush the pan. As soon as the
water in the cistern falls below the entrance of the pipe, air
is sucked in and breaks the siphon. The cistern fills again
and is ready for the next occasion when the chain is pulled.
The larger the bore of the tube and the greater the height
of the cistern above the pan, the more force there is in the
water flushing the pan.

Respiration

Respiration is brought about by the alternate increase and
decrease of pressure in the thorax above and below atmospheric pressure. When the diaphragm descends and the ribs
are raised up by the intercostal muscles, the pressure in the
lungs themselves is reduced below atmospheric pressure. Air
then flows from the region of higher pressure to that of lower
pressure. Expiration takes place when the intrathoracic
pressure becomes greater than atmospheric. The difference
in pressures required to effect this is surprisingly small. In

normal quiet respiration the pressure difference is sufficient to support a column of water about 5 cm high. Compare this with arterial blood pressure which is sufficient to support a column of water 165 cm high.

Intrapleural Pressures

Surrounding the lungs is a double layer of serous membrane called the pleura. The parietal layer is fixed to the chest wall by connective tissue and the visceral layer to the surface of the lung. The two layers are separated by a thin layer of fluid which acts as a lubricant so that the lung can expand and contract without friction. If a needle connected to a 'U' tube manometer is inserted into the space between the layers, the intrapleural space, it is discovered that the pressure in the space is considerably less than atmospheric. It is increased and decreased with inspiration and expiration but remains less than atmospheric at all times. This is sometimes referred to as the 'negative pressure' of the intrapleural space, which, though a contradiction in terms, is quite acceptable as it conveys very well the fact that there is always a suction between the two layers.

There is a good reason why this negative pressure exists. The lung tissue itself is of a balloon-like nature and tends to collapse. The thoracic cage is comparatively rigid. Between the tendency to collapse on one hand, and the tendency to remain rigid on the other, a tension is built up between the two layers of pleura. Because the lung tissue is soft it is prevented from collapsing by this tension or negative pressure. If air enters this space, either by design as in artificial pneumothorax or because of disease as in spontaneous pneumothorax, the tension holding out the lung is destroyed and it collapses.

Artificial Pneumothorax Machines

Some of the most efficient pneumothorax machines utilize the siphon principle. As water flows from one bottle into another the air in the second bottle is pushed out by the incoming water. The displaced air can be conducted along tubing and inserted into a patient's intrapleural space with the aid of a special needle. The delivery tube is connected to a 'U' tube water manometer. This is clipped off and out of action while the air is actually flowing but can be put into action at any moment so that the pressure in the intrapleural space can be ascertained at any stage during the procedure. Usually no more air is allowed to enter than will allow the lung to collapse under its own tendency. Forcible collapsing of the lung compresses it against the mediastinum and may embarrass the heart.

Exercises

1. Calculate the total pressure exerted on a box measuring 60 cm long, 60 cm wide, and 40 cm tall when it is lying under water at a depth sufficient to cause an average pressure of 250 g per sq. cm.

2. What area must a safety valve weighing 1 kg have in order for it to blow when the pressure reaches 2 kg per sq. cm?

3. A careless nurse allows a box weighing 6 kg to fall on the safety valve of a hot water sterilizer and fails to remove it. If the internal area of the valve is 1 sq. cm and is supposed to blow when the pressure reaches 1500 g per sq. cm, what will be the pressure when it actually blows? Is this within the safety limit if the boiler has been tested to 3 kg per sq. cm?

4. Given that the barometric pressure falls 2·5 cm for every 274 m of height, calculate the height of a mountain if the pressure at its foot is 770 mm and at the top is 695 mm.

5. What will the temperature of bottles of saline be during sterilization at a pressure of 5 lb per sq. in.? What will happen if the pressure is suddenly reduced to atmospheric?

6. What will be the barometric pressure at the foot of a mountain if it is 652·5 mm at its summit and the mountain is 959 m high?

17
Graphs

GRAPHS are a means of showing relationships in a pictorial fashion instead of in words or figures. A simple type of graph is the bar or line graph used to show differences in such things as quantity, length, weight, area, volume or practically anything else. Nurses are familiar with this type of graph in the form of intake and output charts. A record is kept of everything fluid that passes into the patient's body whether it is taken orally, rectally or by injection and entered under *intake*. All urine, vomit, haemorrhage and discharge is measured and recorded under *output*. Each day the amounts are totalled thus:

Mr Jones, 17 October

Intake			Output		
Hour		*ml*	*Hour*		*ml*
07.00	tea	140			
08.00	tea	280	07.00	urine	350
08.00	medicine	30	10.00	urine	240
11.00	water	300	11.00	drainage	426
14.00	tea	150	14.00	urine	228
17.00	tea	280	18.00	urine	142
20.00	stout	300	22.00	urine	144
23.00	milk	150			
	Total	1630		Total	1530

The following day a fresh sheet is made out and so it

continues as long as a record is required. Succeeding days may show totals like this:

	Intake ml	Output ml
17	1734	1495
18	2102	1704
19	1591	1000
20	1846	1903
21	2272	1780
22	1875	1648
23	1875	1761
24	2000	2000

In some hospitals this may be regarded as sufficient but it is usual to turn this information into a pictorial record so that it can be seen at a glance how intake and output compare with each other, which is brought up to date each morning. This pictorial record is a **bar graph** and looks like Graph 1.

There are three essentials of any type of graph. Without them a graph is unintelligible to everyone except the person who made it. The poorer types of advertisement sometimes attempt to gull the public by exhibiting the sort of thing shown below. It is arrant nonsense of course, because the graph tells one nothing. It cannot do so. It is meaningless.

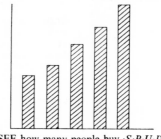

SEE how many people buy ·S·P·U·D·

The next illustration shows the three essential features of a bar graph.

(1) There must be a vertical scale representing quantity.

(2) There must be a horizontal scale representing date.

(3) There must be a key whenever two or more things are represented on a graph.

Bar graphs can be drawn on plain paper as in Graph 1 but it saves considerable work and possibility of error if

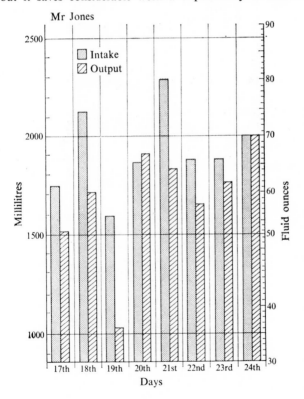

GRAPH 1

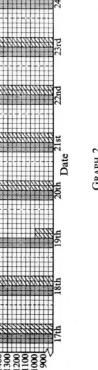

GRAPH 2

squared paper is used. Plain paper has to be ruled with parallel vertical and horizontal lines and all this is done ready for use on squared paper. All that remains to be done is to adapt the existing lines to convenient vertical and horizontal scales.

A vertical line is drawn towards the left of the paper leaving enough room to be able to write between the line and the edge of the paper. A convenient number of squares are counted off and each small square represents a definite quantity. In Graph 2, the vertical line represents millilitres on the left and ounces on the right. Each small square represents 100 ml.

A horizontal line is similarly drawn leaving sufficient room for writing, and this stands for successive days. Every five small squares represents one day. Into this chart is fitted the information gathered each day.

On the 17th (using the previous intake and output record), intake was 1734 ml and output 1495 ml. To represent these quantities on the graph squares are marked out in proportion to the quantity of fluid taken. Do not forget that the base line of 0 ml is not shown so that only quantities in excess of 800 ml can be indicated on the chart. Alongside the output for the day is similarly indicated. The former column is shaded differently to the latter or blocked out in a different colour to distinguish it. In this example horizontal lines are used for intake and diagonal lines for output.

This is repeated each day as the information is gathered and any observer can see all at a glance for the whole of the recorded period.

Another type of graph is the continuous graph used mainly in nursing in the form of temperature and pulse charts. This type of graph shows the inter-relationship of two different things simultaneously. In the case of the temperature charts it shows the relationship between temperature and time. Each spot on the graph shows two things: (a) the temperature of the patient, and (b) the time the temperature was taken. Successive spots give a clear indication of the 'ups' and

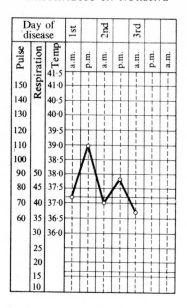

GRAPH 3

Modern temperature charts are designed to be able to provide a lot of information beyond the temperature. This chart is scaled for Celsius and graphs of the pulse and respiration could also be included on it.

'downs' over a period. This gives immediately a clear impression to an observer which a simple written list could never do. The lines drawn connecting the spots make it clearer still.

The same essentials are required for this type of graph as for the bar graph, namely a vertical scale, a horizontal scale, and a key when more than one set of spots are used on the same graph. Squared paper is a useful aid and the temperature charts in use in every hospital are simply a special type of squared paper adapted for that particular form of graph.

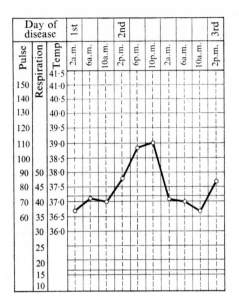

GRAPH 4

*Most temperature charts are so arranged that different
time intervals can be used. This sheet is being used as a
'4-hourly' chart*

The vertical and horizontal scales are already marked off
and space is left for much additional information relevant
to any particular patient.

The successive spots marked on a temperature chart are
usually joined by straight lines. The lines represent the lapse
of time between successive spots. This interval may be any
time at all. It is frequently 12 hr, but can be 6-hourly, 4-hourly
or 2-hourly. The commonest in hospitals are morning and
evening charts and 4-hourly charts. The temperature in
between two successive spots is not known definitely but is

inferred to be something in between the temperatures represented by the two spots.

In Graph 3 the first spot represents 37·2°C (99°F) at 06.00 hours on the first day, and the second spot represents 38·8°C (102°F) at 18.00 hours. At 12.00 hours we infer that the temperature was between these two points but we cannot be sure. It could have been something entirely different. If we want to know more accurately we should have to take the temperature at shorter intervals, say 4-hourly. The graph would look something like Graph 4.

This is a good example of the fact that the shorter the interval of time between successive readings, the greater the degree of accuracy obtainable. Sometimes nurses need to have almost a moment to moment account of a patient's condition; for example, during a critical phase such as immediately after an operation when there is a danger of haemorrhage. For this purpose a special type of graph is drawn showing the relationship between pulse rate and time. At 15-min intervals the pulse is counted and recorded. Graph 5 shows a graph constructed on a 15-min basis.

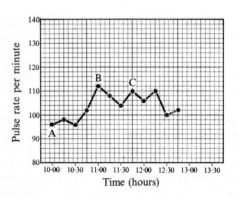

GRAPH 5

The vertical scale represents pulse rate and extends from 80 per minute at its lowest point to 140 at its highest. This is a range of 60 beats and is spread over 30 small squares. Thus each small square represents 2 beats. The horizontal scale is arranged so that each small square represents 3 min so that every fifth square marks off a 15-min period. The spots are placed at the intersections of the relevant vertical and horizontal lines. Spot A represents a pulse rate of 96 because it lies on the horizontal line passing through the scale at 96. It also represents a time of 10.00 hours because it lies on a vertical line passing through 10.00 hours. Similarly spot B represents a pulse rate of 112 at 11.00 hours and spot C 110 at 11.45 hours.

When the interval between recordings is reduced to a negligible period, the spots would be so close together that they would form a continuous line. The individual spots would be unnecessary. Very accurate readings can be taken from continuous line graphs.

An interesting form of continuous line graph is the self recording pressure graphs attached to many autoclaves. These are unusual because they are circular and rotate by clockwork or electricity. A pen is pressed against the graph paper and a line is traced as the paper rotates. The nib is raised or lowered according to the pressure within the auto-clave. Graph 6 shows a simplified diagram of one of these graphs. The radius of the circle takes the place of the vertical scale and the circumference of the circle takes the place of the horizontal scale. In this case the scales are representing pressure in pounds per square inch and time in minutes. The line traced in Graph 6 shows that the autoclave was started at A and a partial vacuum was created until at B the pressure stood at 5 lb per sq. in. This was maintained for 5 min and at C the pressure started to build up until at D it reached 30 lb per sq. in. Between D and E this pressure was maintained for 20 min. From E to F the pressure fell again to 5 lb per sq. in. and was maintained at this pressure until G, i.e. for 20 min.

Thereafter air was admitted until the pressure was atmospheric and the sterilizer was switched off.

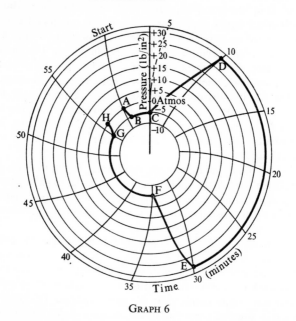

GRAPH 6

In this way a permanent record can be kept every time the autoclave is used and everyone can be sure that the sterilization has been done perfectly.

Now let us construct a graph. A useful one would show the relationship between Celsius and Fahrenheit scales. Instead of having to work out a piece of arithmetic each time we need to convert from one scale to another, all we will need to do is to look up the temperature on one of the scales and see what point corresponds to this on the other scale.

In Graph 7 the horizontal line represents the Celsius scale and shows temperatures between 0° and 100°, a range of 100° over 50 small squares so that each small square represents

2 degrees. The vertical line represents Fahrenheit scale and shows temperatures between 30° and 240° which is 210 degrees

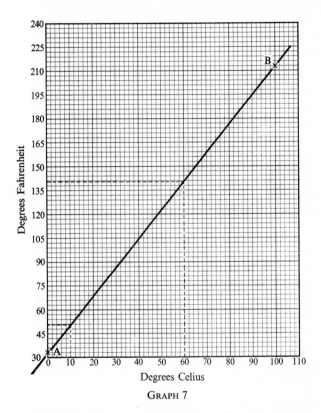

Degrees Celius

GRAPH 7

covering 70 small squares so that each small square represents 3 Fahrenheit degrees.

We know that 0°C equals 32°F because that is the freezing point of water so we can put a cross to show this at A. We also know that the temperature of boiling water is 100° on the Celsius scale and 212° on the Fahrenheit. If we place a cross at B it stands for both these temperatures simultaneously. A line joining A and B completes the graph. The following examples are worked in this fashion.

Look up the temperature 50°F along the vertical scale. A line is extended horizontally from this point to meet the graph line. From the point where it cuts the graph line a line is extended to the horizontal scale and the temperature read where it cuts the horizontal scale. This is the temperature in degrees Celsius, i.e. 10°C. Actual extension lines have been drawn in this case but it is sufficient to place a ruler on the graph and imagine the lines.

The second example shows how to convert Celsius degrees to Fahrenheit. 60°C is located on the horizontal scale. A line is projected from this point to cut the graph. From the point where it cuts the graph a second line is projected horizontally until it meets the vertical scale. At this point the temperature is read off. It is 140°F.

Exercises

1. With the aid of Graph 7 convert the following Celsius degrees to the Fahrenheit scale; 60, 5, 20, 35, 66, 68, 75, 92.

2. Convert the following Fahrenheit degrees to the Celsius scale: 50, 45, 72, 96, 108, 127, 138, 200, 98·4.

3. Check each one of these by arithmetic.

Example: Construct a graph from the following data showing the relationship between age and weight in an average child during the first 4 months of life.

Age in weeks	Weight in lb	Weight in kg
0	7·25	3·29
1	6·75	3·06
2	7·2	3·27
3	7·75	3·52

Age in weeks	Weight in lb	Weight in kg
4	8	3·63
5	8·4	3·81
6	8·75	3·97
7	9·1	4·13
8	9·5	4·31
9	10	4·54
10	10·45	4·74
11	10·9	4·94
12	11·2	5·08
13	11·6	5·26
14	12·2	5·53
15	12·8	5·81
16	13·2	5·99

The vertical line represents weight and extends from 3 kg which is a little below requirements to 6 kg which is a little above. This range of 3 kg extends over 60 small squares so that each square represents 0·05 of a kilogram. The horizontal line stands for age. 16 weeks are represented by 40 small squares so that one week is represented by $2\frac{1}{2}$ small squares.

The information is charted carefully until a series of crosses result. These are joined by straight lines. Point A occurs where '0' on the age line intersects 3·29 kg on the weight line. Point B occurs where '1' on the age line intersects 3·06 kg on the weight line and so on.

From Graph 8 find the following information

1. Did the baby make up her birth weight in 2 weeks?

2. What was the weight at $8\frac{1}{2}$ weeks?

3. How old was the baby when she weighed 3·72 kg?

4. Did she double her birth weight under the observation period?

5. Did the baby lose weight at any time?

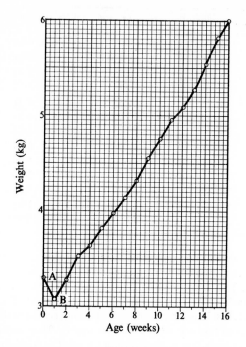

GRAPH 8

Exercises

1. Make a temperature chart using squared paper to include the following:

1st day		2nd day		3rd day		4th day		5th day		6th day		7th day	
a.m.	p.m.	a.m.	p.m.	a.m.	p.m.	a.m.	p.m.	a.m.	p.m.	a.m.	p.m.	a.m.	p.m.
°C 36·4	°C 37·2	°C 36·6	°C 37·4	°C 36·1	°C 37·8	°C 37·2	°C 38·5	°C 37·6	°C 37·6	°C 37	°C 37·5	°C 36·1	°C 37·2

2. Make a temperature chart using squared paper to show the following information:

First day			Second day			Third day		
02·00 hours	06·00 hours	10·00 hours	02·00 hours	06·00 hours	10·00 hours	02·00 hours	06·00 hours	10·00 hours
°F 98·4	°F 98	°F 98·2	°F 102·2	°F 99·4	°F 99	°F 101	°F 99·2	°F 99
14·00 hours	18·00 hours	22·00 hours	14·00 hours	18·00 hours	22·00 hours	14·00 hours	18·00 hours	22·00 hours
°F 99	°F 101·6	°F 102	°F 100·2	°F 102·4	°F 102	°F 99·4	°F 100	°F 100·2

3. Construct a blank for recording the pulse rate at 15-min intervals, in readiness for a patient returning from theatre, to extend over 12 hr.

4. Make a bar graph to show the following intake and output over 1 week:

Day	Intake (ml)	Output (ml)
1	1320	1180
2	1380	1180
3	1200	1240
4	1560	1360
5	1440	1360
6	1140	1240
7	1800	1550

5. Graph 9 is a graph showing pulse and temperature together from the same patient.

(a) What was the temperature and pulse rate at 'A'?

(b) What was temperature and pulse rate at 'B'?

(c) When the temperature was 100°F what was the pulse rate?

(*d*)   When the pulse rate was 100 beats per minute what was the temperature?

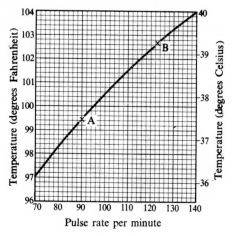

GRAPH 9

6.   Construct a bar graph showing the following rainfall month by month:

January	3·7	February	0·8	March	1·8
April	2	May	3·4	June	1·2
July	1	August	nil	September	0·4
October	3·6	November	2	December	2·2

(*a*)   What was the total rainfall?
(*b*)   What was the average rainfall?
(*c*)   Which was the wettest month?
(*d*)   Which was the driest month?

7.   Draw a graph to show the following information which is the acidity found in a normal stomach by means of a Fractional Test Meal. Specimens were taken at 15-min intervals for $2\frac{1}{2}$ hr.

Fasting	20 ml	90 min	30 ml
15 min	5 ml	105 min	25 ml
30 min	15 ml	120 min	30 ml
45 min	30 ml	135 min	25 ml
60 min	35 ml	150 min	20 ml
75 min	36 ml		

Join the points plotted by a curved line.

8. Draw a graph showing the relationship of weight and age in an average male of height 5 ft 8 in. using the following information:

Age	Weight (kg)	Age	Weight (kg)
16	61·7	32	69·9
18	63·5	34	70·3
20	65·3	36	70·7
22	66·2	38	71·2
24	67·1	40	71·7
26	68	42	72·1
28	68·5	44	72·6
30	68·9	46	73

9. On the same graph as the previous question show the following information which is the relationship between age and weight in an average woman of 5 ft 2 in.

Age	Weight (kg)	Age	Weight (kg)
16	50·3	32	55·8
18	51·7	34	56·7
20	52·6	36	57·1
22	53	38	57·6
24	54	40	58·5
26	54·4	42	59
28	54·8	44	59·9
30	55·3	46	60·3

18
Uses of statistics

ALTHOUGH a full treatment of the science of statistics is beyond the scope of this book, a brief study of some of the methods used by statisticians is worthwhile. We often ask or are asked questions with statistical implications. For example: Why do pupils in one school always get better results in examinations than pupils in a similar school down the road? Is poverty still a serious problem? If so, to what extent? Do many old people fail to get a balanced diet because protein foods are so expensive? These and many other matters are frequent topics of discussion. Many opinions are expressed, sometimes cogently, but little information of real value can emerge from such discussion unless reliable facts are available to the participants.

Statistics is partly the science of collecting and summarizing facts which can be expressed in numerical form; it is concerned also with the measurement and comparison of facts to try and discover the existence of significant relationships, to reveal trends and so to assist those charged with responsibility for making estimates or forecasts.

The Normal Curve

If data on a research subject was obtained from the whole of the population of a country, for example information on physical attributes, it would be possible to tabulate the information and arrive at average values for each attribute. Let us consider height. From the mass of information received we would find that most people would be of average height or very near it; the number of people deviating from the average would become progressively smaller as we look towards the extremes of very short and very tall. This is shown in the diagram below.

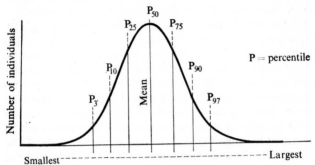

Source: *Documenta Geigy*, Scientific Tables.
Key: 3rd to 97th percentile–94% of all Individuals
     10th to 90th percentile–80% of all individuals
     25th to 75th percentile–50% of all individuals
Normal distribution of body length

The curve shows the normal distribution of the body length of a large number of people. It will be seen that the numbers at each extreme are similar and that the great majority of people are in the middle ranges. This is an example of *the normal curve*.

Statisticians work on the assumption that given a sufficiently large sample the probability is that the distribution of values will follow the distribution shown on a normal curve. In practice it is rarely possible to obtain information from such large numbers of people and it is necessary to take samples, that is, information, from a comparatively small proportion of the populace. If the results of statistical work are to be reliable the opinion of a good cross-section of the population must be obtained.

Special techniques are used to avoid, or to try and avoid any bias which would unfairly influence and therefore invalidate the results of research. Imagine the results of an enquiry aimed at making a forecast of the results of a general election if people having allegiance to only one of the political parties were questioned! Could the findings be free of prejudice? Alternatively, imagine trying to obtain a reliable sample by taking every fifth name in the telephone directory. This would seem, on the surface, to be a good way of obtaining a random sample, but what about the large number of people who cannot afford or who do not want a telephone? A moments reflection will reveal that such a sample would not be representative. Everyone should always examine statistical information very carefully to ascertain the source of information and to see what the compiler is attempting to portray. It should be noted that the word 'population' is often used in statistics to describe a group of people who are the subject of a particular piece of research.

Symbols

A brief description of some of the symbols commonly used in statistics is given below, although few symbols are used in this chapter. They are merely a shorthand method of writing expressions which are very long and cumbersome if written in full.

Σ = the sum (addition) of a series of figures. It is the Greek character—large sigma—the equivalent of our S.

x = the individual items in a series.

$\bar{x}$ = the arithmetic mean.

N or n = total frequencies.

f = frequency.

a = assumed mean.

d = deviations from the assumed mean.

Q = Quartile. The quarters are usually written as Q_1 for the lower quartile ($\frac{1}{4}$) and Q_3 for the upper quartile ($\frac{3}{4}$).

Sources of Information

An adequate amount of information must be gathered before any figures can be scientifically treated and meaningful relationships educed. If the sets of numbers are too small it would be most unwise to draw an inference from the results. At times the information has to be obtained direct from people using techniques such as postal questionnaires or personal interviews; this information is called primary data. Information already available in reports, articles or other published work is called secondary data.

Tabulation

Once the required data has been obtained the groups of facts to be treated are extracted and placed in some order so that they become easier to grasp and manipulate; this process is called tabulation. For example, consider the table below showing the length of time spent in hospital by a hypothetical group of patients.

Number of days spent in hospital by a group of 55 patients

12	20	11	9	8	15	8	5	14	11	21
27	2	17	7	15	10	19	13	17	3	23
3	14	7	11	17	4	13	18	2	15	21
16	17	13	19	14	12	18	6	12	18	22
15	14	6	13	9	16	12	11	25	16	23

It is difficult to see any significance in these figures until they have been rearranged and the frequency of particular numbers can be clearly seen. To achieve this object the numbers have been rearranged in the table below.

Days	Frequency	Days	Frequency	Days	Frequency
1	0	11	4	21	2
2	2	12	4	22	1
3	2	13	4	23	2
4	1	14	4	24	0
5	1	15	4	25	1
6	2	16	3	26	0
7	2	17	4	27	1
8	2	18	3	28	0
9	2	19	2	29	0
10	1	20	1	30	0

Now a definite pattern is beginning to emerge. If we go a step further and arrange the numbers in groups with a suitable class interval an impression can be obtained at a glance.

Number of days in hospital	Number of patients
1 to 4 days	5
5 to 8 days	7
9 to 12 days	11
13 to 16 days	15
17 to 20 days	10
21 to 24 days	5
25 to 28 days	2
Total	55

It is apparent that the class interval selected is four days and that the majority of the hypothetical patients stayed in hospital for 13 to 16 days. The column is reproduced again below with a third column added showing the cumulative frequency. This column is sometimes used to help show at a glance the proportion or percentage above or below a given value.

Number of days in hospital	Number of patients	Cumulative frequency
1 to 4 days	5	5
5 to 8 days	7	12
9 to 12 days	11	23
13 to 16 days	15	38
17 to 20 days	10	48
21 to 24 days	5	53
25 to 28 days	2	55
Total	55	

The numbers in the third column are obtained by means of simple addition of the numbers in the second column, the product each time being placed under cumulative frequency Thus $5 + 7 = 12$, $12 + 11 = 23$, and so on. The table shows, for example, that 23 people stayed in hospital for less than 13 days, whereas only 17 stayed in hospital for more than 16 days. When a table contains a long list of figures a cumulative frequency column can be a very useful asset.

Diagrams

Diagrams of various types are often used in statistics as a simple but effective means of conveying an instant impression of information gleaned from groups of figures. A histogram is a popular form of diagram, in which the areas within blocks represent the frequencies of particular values. If we use our group of 55 patients just once more we can make a histogram showing the length of stay in hospital, as shown on the next page.

Histograms can be used without the ordinate (the vertical line and abscissa (the horizontal line) being drawn if values are written into the blocks. The following histogram is an illustration of the way in which comparisons can be drawn.

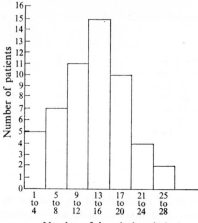

Histogram showing the length of stay in hospital of a group of 55 patients

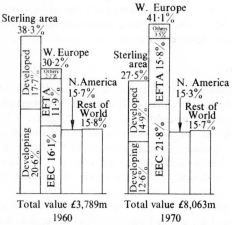

Source: *H. M. Government Fact Sheet* No. 5 (1971)

Britains export markets

Pictograms

These, as the name suggests, are pictorial means of conveying information that are popular with newspapers, magazines and journals. The pictogram below is an example that shows the income tax paid by a single person; a married couple and a married couple with children in 1960.

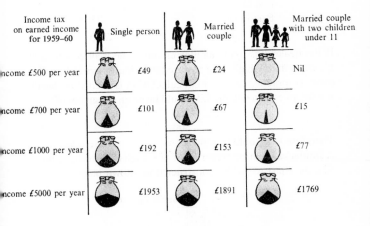

Income tax on earned income for 1959–60	Single person	Married couple	Married couple with two children under 11
Income £500 per year	£49	£24	Nil
Income £700 per year	£101	£67	£15
Income £1000 per year	£192	£153	£77
Income £5000 per year	£1953	£1891	£1769

Source: *Central Office of Information.*

Pie Charts

A pie chart may be used to represent variable quantities, although the number of quantities shown should not be too many if the diagram is to be effective. The chart is based on a circle so all the quantities together will be represented by the whole 360° of the circle. Each quantity is calculated as a proportion of the whole (in terms of a number of degrees) and is shown as a segment of the pie chart. Let us take as an example a nurse who expects to travel about 10,000 miles a year and who is seeking advice on the cost of running a new car. The dealer may give information as follows:

Estimated Annual Cost of Motoring (10,000 miles)

	£
Petrol and oil	140
Tyres and brake maintenance	17
Servicing charges	16
Depreciation	270
Insurance	32
Road tax	25
	£500

If the dealer has many similar enquiries he may construct a pie chart that will give the required information quickly and is easily comprehended. A small calculation is needed to decide the size of each segment. £25 would be given a segment of:

$$25 \times \frac{360}{500} = 18$$

Therefore £25 would be represented by 18° of the circle.
A similar calculation is carried out for each of the other values.
The pie chart would be constructed as shown below.

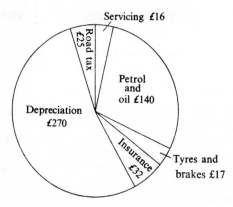

Pie chart showing the cost of motoring 10,000 miles in 1 year.

Bar Diagrams

These also are useful for illustrating information in an effective manner. The bars may be drawn vertically or horizontally, the choice depends on whichever is thought to have the greatest visual impact. The next diagram draws a comparison between five systems of farming in as many counties. All the farms have an approximate level of investment of £200,000. The compilers object is to show the relationship between the value of each farm and the earnings as a percentage of capital invested.

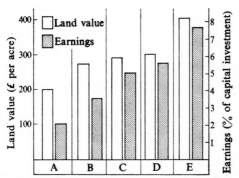

Land values and earnings in: (A) Northumberland, (B) Gloucestershire, (C) Norfolk, (D) Shropshire, and (E) Lincolnshire

Source: *The Daily Telegraph* Financial Column (25 September 71)

It can be quickly seen from the diagram that the return on investment ranges from 2 to 7·5%.

Graphs

Many business people use graphs to show the rate of increase or decrease of their sales as they are particularly suited to this purpose. In a similar way some hospital authorities use them to plot the rates of admission and discharge of their patients. Variables which are measured at regular intervals are known as time series. An example is given in the following table which shows the total number of people attending and the total number passing the State final examinations between February 1967 and February 1971.

Number of student nurses who attended and the number who passed the State final examinations from February 1967 to February 1971

Date of examination		
Year Month	*Number present*	*Number successful*
1967 February	6529	4441
June	6228	4095
October	7454	5118
1968 February	7258	4730
June	6962	4341
October	7973	5315
1969 February	7241	4893
June	6617	4037
October	7870	5100
1970 February	7205	4501
June	6728	4264
October	7269	4594
1971 February	6748	4316

It is not easy to see a definite pattern by simply looking at the figures, but if they are shown on a graph they have meaning so now we will plot them onto a graph.

Obviously there is little hope of plotting numbers to the nearest unit on a graph of this size, so the figures have become approximate to the nearest fifty. However, the graph serves its purpose of giving an immediate overall view of the increase and decrease of attendance and pass rates over the 4-year period.

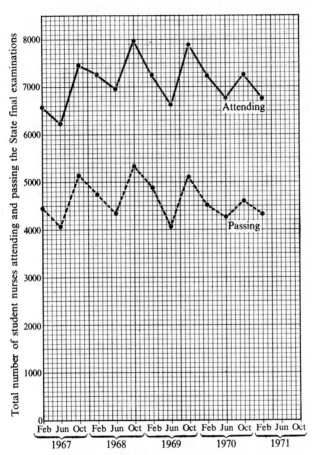

Source : Annual Reports of the General Nursing Council for England and Wales

Averages

We have seen how tabulation and diagrammatic presentation can aid the understanding of available data. Now we shall see how the determination of averages provides further description of a collection of figures and helps to bring out the salient points. The arithmetic mean, median and mode are the averages most commonly used in statistics; the harmonic and geometric averages belong to a more advanced study of the subject.

An arithmetic mean is obtained by dividing the sum of a series of values by the number of values. This is the measure to which most people refer when they speak of 'average'.

Example: Eight people pay weekly rent of £5·25; £6·40; £8·50; £10·35; £9·70; £7·80; £6·80; and £10·00 respectively. What is the mean amount of rent?
The total paid is:

$$
\begin{array}{r}
£ \\
5·25 \\
6·40 \\
8·50 \\
10·35 \\
9·50 \\
7·80 \\
6·80 \\
10·00 \\
\hline
£64·80
\end{array}
$$

Therefore the arithmetic mean will be

$$\frac{£64·80}{8} = \textbf{£8·10}$$

When a number of values recur a frequency table can be constructed before the arithmetic mean is calculated.

Example: During a 31-day period a casualty department treats numbers of patients for minor injuries, as shown in the following table.

Day	No.	Day	No.	Day	No.	Day	No.	Day	No.	Day	No.
1	55	6	23	11	23	16	25	21	58	26	23
2	25	7	70	12	44	17	18	22	18	27	18
3	18	8	18	13	18	18	20	23	44	28	55
4	21	9	25	14	55	19	23	24	20	29	47
5	32	10	21	15	47	20	32	25	21	30	20
										31	23

What is the arithmetic mean?

The numbers are first arranged according to frequency, the number of days is then multiplied by the respective frequency to obtain the total number of patients treated. Note the symbols (x), (f) and $(x \times f)$; these signify the number of items (x) and the frequency (f).

Number of incidents per day (x)	Frequency (number of days) (f)	Total number of incidents ($x \times f$)
18	6	108
20	3	60
21	3	63
23	5	115
25	3	75
32	2	64
44	2	88
47	2	94
55	3	165
59	1	59
70	1	70
	31	961

arithmetic mean $= \dfrac{961}{31} = 31.$

Therefore the average number of injuries treated each day over a 31-day period was 31.

A short method of finding the arithmetic mean can be used when the number of values is large. The first step is to arrange the values in ascending order and then the frequency of each number is written in a parallel column. From a study of the numbers so displayed an estimate of the probable arithmetic mean is made. If the values in the first column involve a range, a third column is written giving the mid-point of each range. Thus for a range of 1 to 9 years the mid-point will be 5 years. If decimal values would be inappropriate ranges such as 1 to 10 should be avoided. Having progressed so far, another column is added for deviations from the assumed mean; for this purpose a class interval can be used if all the values are in proportion to each other.

Example: Determine the average age of a group of 100 nurses.

Age range (years)	No. of nurses (f)	Mid-point (x)	Deviation (d)	Deviation class interval $\left(\dfrac{d}{c}\right)$	frequency $\times \dfrac{d}{c}$ $\left(f \times \dfrac{d}{c}\right)$
21 to 25	24	23	-15	-3	-72
26 to 30	10	28	-10	-2	-20
31 to 35	12	33	-5	-1	-12
*36 to 40	14	38	0	0	0
41 to 45	14	43	$+5$	$+1$	-14
46 to 50	8	48	$+10$	$+2$	$+16$
51 to 55	11	53	$+15$	$+3$	$+33$
56 to 60	7	58	$+20$	$+4$	$+28$
	100				$+91$
					-104
					-13

* The assumed mean = 38 years

Note:

1. The first two columns are self evident. The mid-point values of each range in the first column have been placed in the third column (*x*).

2. Columns 3 (*x*), 4 (*d*) and (5 (*d/c*) are really all related. To obtain the deviation column the assumed mean has been deducted from each mid-point value. As there is a class interval of 5 the numbers can be reduced still further by dividing each deviation by 5.

3. The last column is obtained by multiplying the number of nurses in each range by *d/c*, e.g. 24 × −3 = −72. This is obviously easier and quicker than multiplying 24 × 23. The whole point of obtaining columns *d* and *d/c* is to reduce the amount of tedious counting.

4. Now that column *f(d/c)* has been completed, add and subtract the numbers as indicated by the signs. Thus: +91 − 104 = −13.

5. The true arithmetic mean is found by means of the following formula:

$$\bar{x} = a + \left(\frac{c \times \sum f \frac{d}{c}}{n} \right)$$

Key: $\bar{x}$ = arithmetic mean: *a* = assumed mean, *c* = class interval.

$\sum$ = the sum of: *f* = frequency, *d* = deviation.

$\sum f \frac{d}{c}$ = the sum of frequency multiplied by (deviation divided by class interval)

substituting numbers for the symbols we have:
true arithmetic mean

$$= 38 + \left(\frac{5 \times -13}{100} \right) \text{ years } = 38 + \left(\frac{-65}{100} \right)$$
$$= 38 + (-0.65) = 38 - 0.65$$

therefore the mean
$$= 37.35 \text{ years.}$$

The Median

Sometimes the arithmetic mean can be influenced by a very high or a very low figure in a series. Consider for example fifteen men whose weekly earnings amount to the following sums: £27; £30; £32; £32; £32; £32; £33; £33; £34; £34; £35; £35; £36; £40 and £45. The arithmetic mean would be

$$\frac{\overset{102}{\underset{3}{510}}}{15} = £34$$

This seems to be a reasonable average, but if, in addition, another four men whose earnings are £100; £160; £180 and £190 a week are considered the arithmetic mean would be

$$\frac{1140}{19} = £60$$

The average has obviously been distorted by the high earnings of only four men.

To help correct the distorting effect of extreme values on an arithmetic mean the median value can be selected. The median (or middle) value is easily obtained when there is an odd number of values in a series; in such cases there will be an equal number of values above and below the median value. It is obtained by the formula

$$\frac{N + 1}{2}$$

where N equals the number of values. Thus in the above example the median value will be:

$$\frac{19 + 1}{2} = \frac{20}{2} = 10$$

The tenth value in the series is £34. If the list is checked we will find nine values above and nine values below the median:

27: 30 :32: 32: 32: 32: 33: 33: 34: *34*:

$$\underbrace{\qquad\qquad\qquad\qquad\qquad}_{\text{1 to 9}} \quad \underset{\text{10th}}{\uparrow}$$

$$35: 35: 36: 40: 45: 100: 160: 180: 190.$$

$$\underbrace{}_{\text{11 to 19}}$$

Clearly the median value of £34 is a more accurate portrayal of average earnings than the arithmetic mean of £60.

When there is an even number of values the median is obtained by adding the two middle values and dividing by two. To obtain the median of the numbers 100; 160; 180; and 190, the formula

$$\frac{N + 1}{2}$$

is again used.

$$\frac{4 + 1}{2} = 2 \cdot 5$$

The half indicates that the median is between the second and third value, therefore the median is

$$\frac{160 + 180}{2} = 170$$

If data has been arranged in groups as shown in the table of nurses ages the formula for the median is

$$\frac{N}{2} = \frac{\text{Number of values}}{2}$$

Thus the median age would be $\frac{100}{2} = 50$. That is the age of the fiftieth nurse.

To return to the series of weekly earnings, by taking the division process further we can arrive at the middle values in the ranges above and below the median; these are called quartiles. The first quartile is obtained by the formula

$$\frac{N + 1}{4} = \frac{19 + 1}{4} = 5$$

Therefore the first quartile (Q_1) is the fifth value in the series, which is £32. The third quartile is obtained by the formula

$$\frac{3(N + 1)}{4} = \frac{3(19 + 1)}{4} = \frac{60}{4} = 15$$

Therefore the upper quartile is the fifteenth value, which is £45. Whenever the division yields odd quarters the quartile value is taken to be the nearest whole value. The formulae

$$\frac{N}{4} \text{ and } \frac{3N}{4}$$

are used when grouped data is being considered. Statisticians sometimes take these calculations even further to obtain deciles (tenths) and percentiles (hundredths) using the formulae

$$\frac{N}{10} \text{ and } \frac{N}{100}, \text{ etc.}$$

The Mode

The mode is the most frequently occurring value in a series. This kind of average is particularly useful to clothing and shoe merchants; their average sizes are those for which the demand (and sales) is highest. One more reference to the series of weekly earnings will show that the mode for that series, is £32.

From a study of the averages described and the range of values it is possible for the spread of a series to be observed and measured. Knowledge of the spread, sometimes called scatter or dispersion, examined by the use of techniques which determine, for example, the mean deviation and standard deviation, is helpful to enable statisticians to interpret the available data.

Index Numbers

Before leaving the subject of statistics it is helpful to take a brief look at index numbers. These are the basis of commonly quoted (or misquoted) estimates such as the index of retail prices, popularly known as the cost of living index.

First a base year is selected, the value given to each item in that year will be equated to an index figure of 100. The value of these items in subsequent years is compared with the value in the base year by dividing the new value by the old value and multiplying by 100.

Example

Year	Land value	Index number (*prices relative to 1966*)
1966	£300 an acre	$\frac{300}{300} \times 100 = 100$
1968	£450 an acre	$\frac{450}{300} \times 100 = 150$
1972	£960 an acre	$\frac{960}{300} \times 100 = 320$

It can be seen that the index number is really indicating a percentage increase relative to the value in the base year. A new base year is chosen when the index numbers get too high and become unwieldy.

When a number of items have to be considered as in the index of retail prices, weighting is given to those items considered more important or that occur more frequently.

Example

Item	Price		Percentage increase	Value weight	Product of % increase and weight
	1960	1970			
A	40p	60p	50%	10	500
B	20p	25p	25%	20	500
C	50p	55p	10%	40	400
				70	1400

The product of the last column is divided by the total weighting, to give the weighted percentage change in prices in the 10-year period.

$$\frac{1400}{70} = 20$$

If the 1960 prices are given an index of 100, then the 1970 prices = **120**

This account of statistics has, of necessity, been very brief. However a number of interesting books are available, such as *Use and Abuse of Statistics* by W. J. Reichmann and *Britain in Figures: A Handbook of Social Statistics* by Alan F. Sillitoe (Pelican Original), a further study of this subject is worth undertaking.

Exercises

1. Determine the number of staff in your hospital or unit, as follows;

(*a*) Nursing officers and above.
(*b*) Ward sisters and charge nurses.
(*c*) Staff Nurses and enrolled nurses.
(*d*) Student and pupil nurses.
(*e*) Unqualified staff, e.g. ward orderlies or nursing assistants.

Calculate each of these groups as a percentage of the whole and use the percentages to construct a pie chart. What conclusions can you draw from the chart?

2. Ascertain the age of all the patients in your ward. What is the arithmetic mean age? How does the mean compare with the median age and the mode?

3. Record the length of stay of patients in your ward or unit. Prepare a frequency table, using a suitable class interval and from this draw a histogram. What conclusions can you draw?

4. Find out the average daily cost of keeping patients in your hospital and the average length of stay from the records office. Using these averages as a guide estimate the average cost of the care and treatment given to patients admitted and discharged whilst you were working in one of the wards. Compare the hospital and the ward averages.

5. From a published list of examination results in your school of nursing obtain the marks awarded to all the candidates. Prepare a cumulative frequency table from the figures obtained and plot these onto a graph. From the graph calculate, to the nearest whole mark, the median and quartile scores.

19
Computers and the binary number system

COMPUTERS are being used to an increasing extent in the hospital service and, no doubt, this trend will continue. Many hospitals already have their financial work and other data processed by computers. Some computers are being used as a valuable aid to nursing supervision. In intensive care units, for example, small supervisory systems may be installed to 'watch' body functions such as blood pressure, temperature, respiration, cardiac rhythm (ECG) and brain activity. All these body measurements are fed into a device called a multiplexer and then a type of computer that has a memory bank of about 12,000 words and can process $\frac{3}{4}$ million instructions in one second. An alarm system operates if a patient's condition becomes critical.

Signals fed into a computer are either in digital or analog form. The latter is one which uses a variable voltage or current of electricity to convey a variable signal. For example, if body temperature is being measured then 36·8°C might be represented by 1 volt. A change of temperature in either direction could be represented by an increase or decrease of 1 millivolt for each 0·1°C.

Digital computers can undertake work of much greater complexity, compared with analog computers. Because of this the output from analog computers is often converted, at a rate of about 50,000 signals a second, into digital signals. The output from the digital computer is fed into devices such as television monitors and to magnetic tape for record purposes. A digital system uses a number of on/off states to represent a binary number that is proportional to the measurement being made.

The Binary or Two System

All the work done in this book, so far, has been based on the 'tens' or denary number system. Many other number systems can be used, but for the purpose of computer work the binary or 'two' system is all important. In the binary system the symbols 2, 3, 4, 5, 6, 7, 8 and 9 are not used. All numbers are represented by just two digits, 1 and 0.

Conversion from the Denary to the Binary System

All binary numbers are expressed as a value of two, that is a power of two. To convert a number all that is necessary is to repeatedly divide by two until there is no remainder. At each stage of the division process the number is either equally divided or there is a remainder of one. The binary number is obtained from the collection of remainders, 0 is written when the number is exactly divided.

Example 1: Convert the denary number 251 into a binary number.

	Remainder = binary number	Remainder as (a power of two)
$251 \div 2 = 125$	1	(2^0)
$125 \div 2 = 62$	1	(2^1)
$62 \div 2 = 31$	0	(2^2)
$31 \div 2 = 15$	1	(2^3)
$15 \div 2 = 7$	1	(2^4)
$7 \div 2 = 3$	1	(2^5)
$3 \div 2 = 1$	1	(2^6)
$1 \div 2 = 0$	1	(2^7)

Thus we have as a series of remainders the digits 1 1 1 1 1 0 1 1. These digits represent the binary number and in this form can be recognized by a digital computer as easily as we recognize

251. In the computer circuits 1 would be shown by switching to the 'on' position whereas 0 would be the 'off' position. Note that the digits are written horizontally so that 2^0 is on the right and is preceded by 2^1; 2^2 and so on, in the same way that units, tens and hundreds are written in the denary system.

Example 2: Convert the denary number 39 into a binary number

		Remainder
$39 \div 2 =$	19	1
$19 \div 2 =$	9	1
$9 \div 2 =$	4	1
$4 \div 2 =$	2	0
$2 \div 2 =$	1	0
$1 \div 2 =$	0	1

Therefore the denary number 39 = the binary number 1 0 0 1 1 1.

Conversion to the Denary Scale from the Binary Scale

The binary number is a row of digits that indicates the powers of two in a progressive manner, starting from the digit on the right. Thus the binary number 11111011 is considered in the following order:

Binary number		*Denary equivalent*
1	$\times 2^0 =$	1
1	$\times 2^1 =$	2
0	$\times 2^2 =$	0
1	$\times 2^3 =$	8
1	$\times 2^4 =$	16
1	$\times 2^5 =$	32
1	$\times 2^6 =$	64
1	$\times 2^7 =$	128
$\therefore$ 11111011	$=$	**251**

Addition

Computers can easily add and subtract by using binary numbers, although the rules appear to be slightly different. The rules to remember are:

$$1st \quad 0 + 0 = 0$$
$$2nd \quad 1 + 0 = 1$$
$$3rd \quad 1 + 1 = 10$$

Care must be taken not to confuse 10 in the third rule with ten in the denary system. As we can only count up to two, $1 + 1 = 0$ with 1 carried over to the next position. The principle is the same that is used when we add nine and one in the denary system; the sum is ten so we place 0 in the units position and carry 1 over to the tens position.

Example

Denary number		Binary number
50	=	110010
+44	=	+101100
94		1011110

To check the answer we can convert 1011110 back to the denary system.

$$0 \times 2^0 = 0$$
$$1 \times 2^1 = 2$$
$$1 \times 2^2 = 4$$
$$1 \times 2^3 = 8$$
$$1 \times 2^4 = 16$$
$$0 \times 2^5 = 0$$
$$1 \times 2^6 = 64$$
$$\overline{94}$$

Therefore the denary number 94 = the binary number 1011110.

Subtraction

The rules for subtraction are:

$$\text{1st} \quad 1 - 1 = 0$$
$$\text{2nd} \quad 10 - 1 = 1$$
$$\text{3rd} \quad 1 - 0 = 1$$

When looking at the second rule it must be remembered that the digit on the left is twice the value of the digit to the right. As the (2^0) column is empty, as indicated by the nought, a digit is borrowed from the next highest column (2^1), therefore $10 - 1 = 1$. If this is still not clear think in terms of powers of 2, e.g.

$$\underbrace{2^1 - 2^0}_{\text{Binary}} = \underbrace{2 - 1 = 1}_{\text{Denary}}$$

Example:

Denary number	*Binary number*
54	110110
−49	− 110001
——	———
5	000101 = 101 as the noughts on the left can be ignored

Once again we can check the answer by converting back to the denary system

$$1 \times 2^0 = 1$$
$$0 \times 2^1 = 0$$
$$1 \times 2^2 = \frac{4}{5}$$

The binary system is not difficult once the principles have been grasped. Computers certainly operate at a tremendous speed using binary numbers. When calculations have been completed the output from the computer may take the form of 'hard copy' from a teleprinter or lineprinter, a view of the answer on a television screen, or the answers may be produced on punched cards, paper tape or magnetic tape.

Exercises

1. Convert the following denary numbers to the binary scale:

(*a*) 54;   (*b*) 47;   (*c*) 23;   (*d*) 35;   (*e*) 143.

2. Convert these binary numbers to the denary scale:

(*a*) 11011;   (*b*) 10001;   (*c*) 110101;   (*d*) 110;
(*e*) 101010101.

3. Add the following numbers and express the answers in the denary scale.

         (*a*)   110011 + 101110 + 110001.
         (*b*)   101 + 1011 + 10000.
         (*c*)   1001 + 1101 + 100110.

4. Subtract the following and express the answers in the denary scale.

         (*a*)   100101 − 10101.
         (*b*)   110110 − 101000.
         (*c*)   110011 − 11101.

Appendix:
Useful tables

Metric Weights

1000 micrograms	=	1 milligram
10 milligrams	=	1 centigram
10 centigrams	=	1 decigram
10 decigrams	=	1 gramme
10 grammes	=	1 decagram
10 decagrams	=	1 hectogram
10 hectograms	=	1 kilogram
1000 kilograms	=	1 tonne

Metric Capacity

10 centimils	=	1 decimil
10 decimils	=	1 mil (1 millilitre)
10 millilitres	=	1 centilitre
10 centilitres	=	1 decilitre
10 decilitres	=	1 litre
10 litres	=	1 decalitre
10 decalitres	=	1 hectolitre

Domestic Equivalents (Approximate)

1 teaspoon	=	5 ml
1 dessertspoon	=	10 ml
1 tablespoon	=	20 ml
1 sherryglass	=	60 ml
1 teacup	=	142 ml
1 breakfastcup	=	230 ml
1 tumbler	=	285 ml

Definitions

A dietetic Calorie is the amount of heat required to raise the temperature of 1 litre (approximately 1000 cm³) of water 1°C.

A British Thermal Unit is the amount of heat required to raise the temperature of 1 pound of water 1°F.

1 Therm equals 100,000 British Thermal Units

1 British Thermal Unit equals ¼ dietetic Calorie

1 Therm equals 25,200 dietetic Calories

Calorie Value of Foodstuffs

1 gramme of fat will produce 9 Calories

1 gramme of protein will produce 4 Calories

1 gramme of carbohydrate will produce 4 Calories

1 ounce of fat will produce 250 Calories

1 ounce of protein will produce 120 Calories

1 ounce of carbohydrate will produce 120 Calories

Weights and Heights

Average Weight and Height of Children and Young People

Boys		Age	Girls	
Weight (kg)	Height (cm)		Weight (kg)	Height (cm)
3·4	50·6	Birth	3·36	50·2
10·07	75·2	1 year	9·75	74·2
12·56	87·5	2 years	12·29	86·6
14·61	96·2	3 years	14·42	95·7
16·51	103·4	4 years	16·42	103·2
18·89	110·0	5 years	18·58	109·4
21·91	117·5	6 years	21·09	115·9
24·54	124·1	7 years	23·68	122·3
27·26	130·0	8 years	26·35	128·0
29·94	135·5	9 years	28·94	132·9
32·61	140·3	10 years	31·89	138·6
35·2	144·2	11 years	35·74	144·7
38·28	146·6	12 years	39·74	151·9
42·18	155·0	13 years	44·95	157·1
48·81	162·7	14 years	49·17	159·6
54·48	167·8	15 years	51·48	161·1
58·83	171·6	16 years	53·07	162·2
61·78	172·7	17 years	54·02	162·5
63·05	174·5	18 years	54·39	162·5

Average Weight of Adults aged 30

Height (cm)	Weight (kg)		
	Small build	Medium build	Large build
WOMEN			
152·5	48·5	53·9	60·7
157·5	51·2	56·6	63·9
162·5	53·9	59·8	67·5
167·5	57·1	63·4	71·6
172·5	60·2	67·0	75·7
178·0	63·4	70·2	78·9
MEN			
167·5	58·4	64·8	72·9
172·5	61·6	68·4	77·0
177·5	65·7	72·9	82·0
183	70·7	78·4	87·9
188	75·7	83·8	94·2

The following tables are included mainly for interest, it is unlikely that nurses will need to refer to these tables very often, if at all.

Avoirdupois Weight

16 drams	= 1 ounce (437·5 grains)
16 ounces	= 1 pound (7000 grains)
14 pounds	= 1 stone
2 stones	= 1 quarter
4 quarters	= 1 hundredweight (cwt)
20 cwt	= 1 ton

Apothecaries' Weight

20 grains	= 1 scruple
3 scruples	= 1 drachm
8 drachms	= 1 ounce (480 grains)
12 ounces	= 1 pound (5760 grains)

Apothecaries' Fluid Measure

$$
\begin{aligned}
60 \text{ minims} &= 1 \text{ fluid drachm} \\
8 \text{ drachms} &= 1 \text{ fluid ounce} \\
20 \text{ ounces} &= 1 \text{ pint} \\
2 \text{ pints} &= 1 \text{ quart} \\
4 \text{ quarts} &= 1 \text{ gallon}
\end{aligned}
$$

Conversion Factors

Milligrams $\times \frac{1}{60}$ = grains
Grammes $\times 15$ = grains
Grammes $\times \frac{1}{28}$ = ounces
Kilograms $\times \frac{11}{5}$ = pounds

Grains $\times 60$ = milligrams
Grains $\times \frac{1}{15}$ = grammes
Ounces $\times 28$ = grammes
Pounds $\times \frac{5}{11}$ = kilograms

Millilitres (c.c.) $\times 15$ = minims
Millilitres $\times \frac{2}{7}$ = fluid drachms
Litres $\times 35$ = fluid ounces
Litres $\times \frac{2}{9}$ = gallons
Litres $\times \frac{7}{4}$ = pints

Minims $\times \frac{1}{15}$ = millilitres (c.c.)
Fluid drachms $\times \frac{7}{2}$ = millilitres
Fluid ounces $\times \frac{1}{35}$ = litres
Gallons $\times \frac{9}{2}$ = litres
Pints $\times \frac{4}{7}$ = litres

Approximations

1 millilitre (c.c.) = 15 minims (16·8 minims exactly)
10 millilitres = 150 minims
1 litre = $1\frac{3}{4}$ pints

1 gramme	= 15 grains
1 kilogram	= 2·2 lb
6⅓ kilograms	= 14 lb (1 stone)
1½ grains	= 100 milligrams
$\frac{1}{10}$ grain	= 6 milligrams
$\frac{1}{100}$ grain	= 0·65 milligrams (or just over ½ mg)
1 grain	= 65 milligrams

Equivalent Doses

These equivalents are not accurate enough for use when making up quantities of drugs.

Grains	Milligrams	Grains	Milligrams
15	1000	$\frac{1}{10}$	6
12	800	$\frac{1}{12}$	5
10	600	$\frac{1}{15}$	4
8	500	$\frac{1}{20}$	3
7½	450	$\left.\frac{1}{24}\right\}$	
6	400	$\left.\frac{1}{25}\right\}$	2·5
5	300	$\frac{1}{30}$	2
4	250	$\frac{1}{40}$	1·5
3	200	$\frac{1}{50}$	1·25
2½	150	$\frac{1}{60}$	1
2	125	$\left.\frac{1}{75}\right\}$	
1½	100	$\left.\frac{1}{80}\right\}$	0·8
1¼	75	$\frac{1}{100}$	0·6
1	60	$\left.\frac{1}{120}\right\}$	
¾	50	$\left.\frac{1}{130}\right\}$	0·5
⅗	40	$\left.\frac{1}{150}\right\}$	
½	30	$\left.\frac{1}{160}\right\}$	0·4
⅖	25	$\frac{1}{200}$	0·3
⅓	20	$\frac{1}{240}$	0·25
¼	15	$\left.\frac{1}{300}\right\}$	
⅕	12·5	$\left.\frac{1}{320}\right\}$	0·2
⅙	10	$\frac{1}{400}$	0·15
⅛	7·5	$\left.\frac{1}{480}\right\}$	
		$\left.\frac{1}{500}\right\}$	0·125
		$\frac{1}{600}$	0·1

Millilitres	Minims	Minims	Millilitres
10	150	100	6·0
9	135	90	5·4
8	120	80	4·8
7	105	70	4·2
6	90	60	3·6
5	75	50	3·0
4	60	40	2·4
3	45	30	1·8
2	30	20	1·2
1	15	10	0·6
0·9	13·5	9	0·54
0·8	12·0	8	0·48
0·7	10·5	7	0·42
0·6	9·0	6	0·36
0·5	7·5	5	0·30
0·4	6·0	4	0·24
0·3	4·5	3	0·18
0·2	3·0	2	0·12
0·1	1·5	1	0·06

Answers to questions

Answers to questions

Chapter 1, page 3

(*1*) 80.   (*2*) 16.   (*3*) 21.   (*4*) 9.   (*5*) 39.   (*6*) 18.   (*7*) 6.

page 7

(*1*) b, d, f.   (*2*) b, c, e.   (*3*) a, b, d.   (*4*) (a) $2 \times 2 \times 3$;
(b) 2×7; (c) 5×7; (d) 2×19; (e) $2 \times 3 \times 23$;
(f) $2 \times 2 \times 5 \times 19$; (g) $2 \times 2 \times 3 \times 7 \times 11$;
(h) $3 \times 5 \times 5 \times 7$.

Chapter 2, page 10

(*1*) ii.   (*2*) viii.   (*3*) v.   (*4*) xvii.   (*5*) xxi.   (*6*) xxviii.   (*7*) xxx.
(*8*) xxix.   (*9*) xviii.   (*10*) xxxvi.   (*11*) xli.   (*12*) xl.   (*13*) xlviii.
(*14*) lv.   (*15*) lix.   (*16*) 2.   (*17*) 4.   (*18*) 8.   (*19*) 40.   (*20*) 60.
(*21*) 7.   (*22*) 14.   (*23*) 38.   (*24*) 24.   (*25*) 15.   (*26*) 48.   (*27*) 88.
(*28*) 16.   (*29*) 51.   (*30*) 22.

Chapter 3, page 14

(*1*) $\frac{9}{16}$.   (*2*) $\frac{2}{3}$.   (*3*) $\frac{3}{7}$.   (*4*) $\frac{10}{11}$.   (*5*) —.   (*6*) $\frac{1}{16}$.   (*7*) $\frac{3}{16}$.
(*8*) $\frac{5}{16}$.   (*9*) $\frac{5}{8}$.   (*10*) $\frac{1}{2}$.   (*11*) $\frac{1}{4}$.   (*12*) $\frac{1}{20}$.   (*13*) $\frac{1}{4}$.   (*14*) $\frac{3}{10}$.
(*15*) $\frac{3}{4}$.   (*16*) $\frac{4}{5}$.   (*17*) $\frac{3}{5}$.   (*18*) $\frac{7}{20}$.   (*19*) $\frac{1}{3}$.   (*20*) $\frac{2}{3}$.   (*21*) $\frac{1}{12}$.
(*22*) $\frac{5}{18}$.   (*23*) 40p.   (*24*) 50p.   (*25*) £1·75.   (*26*) 25p.   (*27*) £1·25.
(*28*) 40 sec.   (*29*) 55 sec.   (*30*) 2 in.   (*31*) 7 in.
(*32*) 5 furlongs or 1100 yards.   (*33*) 15 cwt.

page 18

(*1*) $\frac{5}{10}, \frac{7}{14}, \frac{11}{22}, \frac{20}{40}$.   (*2*) $\frac{6}{8}, \frac{12}{16}, \frac{6}{8}, \frac{9}{12}$.   (*3*) $\frac{6}{10}, \frac{15}{25}, \frac{21}{35}, \frac{36}{60}$.
(*4*) $\frac{15}{24}, \frac{30}{48}, \frac{10}{16}, \frac{45}{72}$.   (*5*) $\frac{1}{3}$.   (*6*) $\frac{1}{5}$.   (*7*) $\frac{1}{3}$.   (*8*) $\frac{1}{3}$.   (*9*) $\frac{2}{5}$.   (*10*) $\frac{4}{5}$.
(*11*) $\frac{3}{4}$.   (*12*) $\frac{5}{16}$.   (*13*) $\frac{1}{4}$.   (*14*) $\frac{7}{24}$.   (*15*) $\frac{3}{8}$.   (*16*) $\frac{2}{13}$.   (*17*) $\frac{1}{2}$.
(*18*) $\frac{1}{4}$.   (*19*) $\frac{3}{8}$.   (*20*) $\frac{3}{4}$.   (*21*) $\frac{1}{4}$.   (*22*) $\frac{1}{8}$.   (*23*) $\frac{1}{100}$.   (*24*) $\frac{1}{20}$.
(*25*) $\frac{1}{50}$.   (*26*) $\frac{1}{20}$.   (*27*) $\frac{1}{3}$.   (*28*) $\frac{1}{2}$.   (*29*) $\frac{1}{4}$.   (*30*) $\frac{1}{6}$.   (*31*) $\frac{1}{6}$.
(*32*) $\frac{1}{6}$.   (*33*) $\frac{1}{100}$.   (*34*) $\frac{1}{4}$.   (*35*) $\frac{1}{3}$.   (*36*) $\frac{1}{20}$.   (*37*) $\frac{2}{3}$.   (*38*) $\frac{3}{8}$.

page 20

(*1*) $2\frac{1}{2}$.   (*2*) $1\frac{1}{4}$.   (*3*) $2\frac{1}{3}$.   (*4*) $1\frac{3}{5}$.   (*5*) $2\frac{3}{4}$.   (*6*) 6.   (*7*) $2\frac{7}{11}$.
(*8*) $2\frac{4}{7}$.   (*9*) $2\frac{1}{3}$.   (*10*) $3\frac{5}{9}$.

page 21

(*1*) $\frac{4}{3}$.   (*2*) $\frac{5}{3}$.   (*3*) $\frac{11}{4}$.   (*4*) $\frac{25}{4}$.   (*5*) $\frac{35}{8}$.   (*6*) $\frac{57}{8}$.   (*7*) $\frac{37}{10}$.
(*8*) $\frac{43}{10}$.   (*9*) $\frac{65}{7}$.   (*10*) $\frac{517}{100}$.

Chapter 4, page 26

(1) $\frac{5}{7}$. *(2)* $\frac{7}{9}$. *(3)* $\frac{8}{9}$. *(4)* $\frac{3}{4}$. *(5)* 1. *(6)* $\frac{2}{3}$. *(7)* $\frac{1}{2}$. *(8)* $\frac{7}{10}$.
(9) $\frac{8}{15}$. *(10)* $\frac{17}{20}$. *(11)* $\frac{1}{2}$. *(12)* $\frac{1}{12}$. *(13)* $1\frac{1}{18}$. *(14)* $\frac{7}{8}$. *(15)* $\frac{5}{7}$.
(16) $2\frac{1}{5}$. *(17)* $\frac{9}{16}$. *(18)* $1\frac{2}{5}$. *(19)* $1\frac{11}{18}$. *(20)* $\frac{3}{8}$. *(21)* $\frac{35}{36}$.
(22) $\frac{1}{4}$. *(23)* $1\frac{1}{10}$. *(24)* $\frac{13}{21}$. *(25)* $\frac{34}{75}$.

page 28

(1) $4\frac{3}{4}$. *(2)* $6\frac{3}{5}$. *(3)* $1\frac{2}{3}$. *(4)* $4\frac{5}{6}$. *(5)* $7\frac{11}{12}$. *(6)* $7\frac{19}{36}$ *(7)* $2\frac{15}{16}$.
(8) $8\frac{5}{12}$. *(9)* $\frac{2}{15}$. *(10)* $1\frac{3}{5}$. *(11)* $3\frac{3}{8}$. *(12)* $\frac{5}{6}$. *(13)* $6\frac{89}{90}$.

page 29

(1) 9 oz. *(2)* £2·50. *(3)* $5\frac{1}{4}$. *(4)* 5 empty beds. *(5)* $\frac{1}{4}$.
(6) 14 hours. *(7)* 16 minutes.

Chapter 5, page 33

(1) $\frac{1}{8}$. *(2)* $\frac{3}{16}$. *(3)* $\frac{1}{4}$. *(4)* $1\frac{3}{4}$. *(5)* $1\frac{1}{3}$. *(6)* $\frac{1}{6}$. *(7)* 1. *(8)* $\frac{4}{15}$.
(9) $1\frac{5}{7}$. *(10)* $\frac{1}{2}$ litre.

page 34

(1) $\frac{6}{7}$. *(2)* $2\frac{2}{6}$. *(3)* $2\frac{1}{2}$. *(4)* $3\frac{1}{2}$. *(5)* $\frac{5}{9}$. *(6)* 3. *(7)* 4. *(8)* $3\frac{3}{4}$.
(9) $\frac{6}{35}$. *(10)* $\frac{3}{22}$. *(11)* 6. *(12)* $\frac{2}{3}$. *(13)* 2. *(14)* $\frac{1}{4}$. *(15)* 20.
(16) $5\frac{3}{5}$. *(17)* 8. *(18)* $102\frac{2}{3}$. *(19)* $2\frac{4}{9}$. *(20)* $3\frac{3}{4}$.

Chapter 6, page 36

(1) $1\frac{1}{9}$. *(2)* $\frac{9}{14}$. *(3)* $5\frac{1}{2}$. *(4)* $11\frac{2}{3}$. *(5)* $\frac{3}{4}$. *(6)* $\frac{7}{24}$. *(7)* $\frac{19}{22}$.
(8) $\frac{2}{3}$. *(9)* $\frac{8}{9}$. *(10)* $1\frac{1}{3}$. *(11)* 14. *(12)* $\frac{4}{5}$. *(13)* 36 books.
(14) 18p. *(15)* 28 pints. *(16)* 30. *(17)* $\frac{5}{12}$. *(18)* 3 whole splints.
(19) 12 beds. *(20)* 14 rolls; 15p left over; 3 decorations.
(21) $26\frac{1}{4}$ miles. *(22)* £20·40.

Chapter 7, page 39

(1) 0·1. *(2)* 0·3. *(3)* 0·6. *(4)* 0·08. *(5)* 0·2. *(6)* 0·25.

page 41

(1) $5\frac{1}{5}$. *(2)* $2\frac{1}{2}$. *(3)* $3\frac{1}{4}$. *(4)* $\frac{3}{5}$. *(5)* $\frac{3}{50}$. *(6)* $\frac{3}{500}$. *(7)* $4\frac{1}{8}$.
(8) $2\frac{11}{20}$. *(9)* $1\frac{1}{20}$. *(10)* $\frac{1}{2000}$.

page 42

(1) 0·35. *(2)* 0·12. *(3)* 0·3125. *(4)* 0·825. *(5)* 0·28125.
(6) 0·6625 *(7)* 2·65. *(8)* 3·46875. *(9)* 2·825. *(10)* 3·456.

page 46

(1) (a) 7; (b) 17; (c) 0·07; (d) 30·4; (e) 73·2. *(2)* (a) 320;
(b) 1704; (c) 0·7; (d) 100·7 (e) 1310. *(3)* 1·449. *(4)* 18·7.
(5) 96·52. *(6)* 0·584. *(7)* 2·1994. *(8)* 0·913. *(9)* 0·0913.
(10) 0·0913. *(11)* 0·00231. *(12)* 27·4104. *(13)* 2·050642.
(14) 0·421875. *(15)* 65·596. *(16)* 93·5415.

page 48

(*1*) (*a*) 0·05; (*b*) 0·2; (*c*) 0·3. (*2*) (*a*) 0·05; (*b*) 0·125; (*c*) 0·1875; (*d*) 0·15. (*3*) (*a*) 0·1; (*b*) 0·04; (*c*) 0·84; (*d*) 0·001. (*4*) (*a*) 0·9; (*b*) 0·4; (*c*) 4; (*d*) 0·011; (*e*) 300; (*f*) 0·056; (*g*) 3·309; (*h*) 0·04; (*i*) 42·1; (*j*) 50. (*5*) (*a*) 99; 990; 9900; (*b*) 87·9; 879; 8790; (*c*) 6; 60; 600; (*d*) 0·1; 1; 10; (*e*) 6·5; 65; 650; (*f*) 4·08; 40·8; 408; (*g*) 932·8; 9328; 93,280; (*h*) 70·5; 705; 7050; (*i*) 400·2; 4002; 40,020. (*6*) (*a*) 75; 7·5; 0·75; (*b*) 6·232; 0·6232; 0·06232; (*c*) 0·423; 0·0423; 0·00423; (*d*) 0·0025; 0·00025; 0·000025. (*7*) (*a*) 7·2; (*b*) 0·93; (*c*) 0·012; (*d*) 70·08. (*8*) (*a*) $\frac{9}{10}$; (*b*) $\frac{9}{100}$; (*c*) $\frac{1}{4}$; (*d*) $2\frac{1}{4}$; (*e*) $\frac{56}{125}$; (*f*) $2\frac{19}{250}$; (*g*) $\frac{1}{400}$. (*9*) (*a*) 0·0575; (*b*) 0·00648; (*c*) 157·2; (*d*) 49·602; (*e*) 90·712; (*f*) 262·2048. (*10*) (*a*) $0{\cdot}\dot{3}$; (*b*) $0{\cdot}8\dot{3}$; (*c*) $0{\cdot}\dot{1}$; (*d*) $0{\cdot}\dot{2}\dot{7}$; (*e*) $0{\cdot}\dot{1}4285\dot{7}$. (*11*) (*a*) 24,800; (*b*) 276,000 (*c*) 976,000; (*d*) 0·0076; (*e*) 0·88; (*f*) 0·094; (*g*) 0·067. (*12*) 0·225 litre; 2·25 decilitres; 225 millilitres (*13*) 1·505 tons. (*14*) 23 trays. (*15*) £20·274. (*16*) 350 g carbohydrate, 125 g protein, 25 g fat. (*17*) 10 nurses.

Chapter 8, page 53

(*1*) £145. (*2*) £336·85½. (*3*) £213·63. (*4*) £106·49½. (*5*) £56·66 (*6*) £1176·42. (*7*) £489·65 to nearest 1p. (*8*) 45½p. (*9*) £10·70. (*10*) £179·40. (*11*) £145. (*12*) £11·92.

page 56

(*1*) £6·25. (*2*) £50. (*3*) 380 guilders. (*4*) £10. (*5*) 15p a pound (weight). (*6*) £124.

Chapter 9, page 62

(*1*) 1000 mg. (*2*) 1000 ml. (*3*) 3·155 m. (*4*) 0·25 litre. (*5*) 1·5 g. (*6*) 1750 ml. (*7*) 0·04856 litre. (*8*) 1080 ml. (*9*) 15 cm^3. (*10*) 100 ml. (*11*) 62 mg. (*12*) 0·96 litre. (*13*) 0·0459 litre. (*14*) 9600 g. (*15*) 40·364 litres. (*16*) 1·272 g. (*17*) 7 litres, 531 ml. (*18*) 23·54 mg, 0·02354 g. (*19*) 750 μg. (*20*) 0·75 mm.

page 68

(*1*) (*a*) 0·225 kg, 0·495 lb; (*b*) 3·55 kg, 7·81 lb; (*c*) 0·221 kg, 0·4862 lb; (*d*) 1·4 kg; 3·08 lb. (*2*) (*a*) 0·227 kg, 227 g; (*b*) 4·545 kg, 4545 g; (*c*) 1 kg, 1000 g; (*d*) 2·5 kg, 2500 g. (*3*) (*a*) 6 st 4 lb, 7 st $7\frac{3}{5}$ lb, 8 st $11\frac{1}{5}$ lb, 9 st $1\frac{3}{5}$ lb, 9 st $10\frac{2}{5}$ lb 15 st 10 lb; (*b*) $60\frac{2}{3}$ kg, $133\frac{1}{2}$ lb approximately. (*4*) (*i*) 8400 ml;

8·4 litre; (*ii*) 1500 ml, 1·5 litre; (*iii*) 3150 ml, 3·15 litre; (*iv*) 2800 ml, 2·8 litre. (*5*) (*a*) 28, 70, 119, 0·875, 10·5 ml; (*b*) 2·05, 2·57, 16, 14, 28½ fl dr. (*6*) (*a*) 1⅖ fl oz, 3½ fl oz, 52½ fl oz, 17½ fl oz, 13⅛ fl oz; (*b*) 0·57 litre, 0·057 litre, 10·5 ml, 14·3 ml. (*7*) 1·2 g. (*8*) 0·8 g, 1086 mg, 1 lb, 0·75 kg. (*9*) 300 cm³, 0·75 pint; 0·5 litre; 625 ml; 180 fl oz.

page 70

(*1*) (*a*) 37·84 in.; (*b*) 1·32 in.; (*c*) 5·12 in.; (*d*) 1·48 in.; (*e*) 3·4 in.; (*f*) 50·52 in.; (*g*) 0·84 in.; (*h*) 0·56 in.; (*i*) 7·2 in.
(*2*) (*a*) 1050 mm; (*b*) 2200 mm; (*c*) 43·75 mm; (*d*) 562·5 mm; (*e*) 950 mm; (*f*) 72·5 mm; (*g*) 365 mm; (*h*) 1420 mm; (*i*) 1800 mm. (*3*) 90, 55, 87·5 cm. (*4*) (*a*) 143 lb; (*b*) 290·4 lb; (*c*) 105·6 lb; (*d*) 46·2 lb; (*e*) 233·2 lb; (*f*) 72·6 lb; (*g*) 167·2 lb; (*h*) 35·2 lb; (*i*) 114·4 lb. (*5*) (*a*) 33·6 kg; (*b*) 69·5 kg; (*c*) 15 kg; (*d*) 41·8 kg; (*e*) 33·6 kg; (*f*) 17·7 kg; (*g*) 29·9 kg; (*h*) 30·8 kg; (*i*) 9·55 kg. (*6*) (*a*) 49·9 kg; (*b*) 51·7 kg; (*c*) 66·3 kg; (*d*) 89 kg; (*e*) 85·8 kg; (*f*) 95·3 kg. (*7*) 8·1 kg. (*8*) 283·2 mg. (*9*) (*a*) 18·6 oz; (*b*) 7·7 oz; (*c*) 66·85 oz; (*d*) 29·1 oz; (*e*) 22·4 oz; (*f*) 11·2 oz; (*g*) 26·3 oz; (*h*) 19·3 oz; (*i*) 16·5 oz. (*10*) (*a*) 1511 ml; (*b*) 798 ml; (*c*) 941 ml; (*d*) 131 ml; (*e*) 428 ml; (*f*) 117 ml; (*g*) 912 ml; (*h*) 274 ml; (*i*) 2366 ml.

Chapter 10, page 78

(*1*) (*a*) $\frac{1}{100}$, 0·01; (*b*) $\frac{1}{10}$, 0·1; (*c*) $\frac{3}{20}$, 0·15; (*d*) $\frac{1}{5}$, 0·2; (*e*) $\frac{2}{5}$, 0·4; (*f*) $\frac{1}{2}$, 0·5; (*g*) $\frac{3}{4}$, 0·75; (*h*) $\frac{9}{10}$, 0·9. (*2*) (*a*) 1%; (*b*) 5%; (*c*) 24%; (*d*) 35%; (*e*) 9%; (*f*) 96%; (*g*) 75%; (*h*) 87½%. (*3*) (*a*) 30%; (*b*) 75%; (*c*) 42%; (*d*) 1%; (*e*) 66%; (*f*) 25%; (*g*) 30½%; (*h*) 39·3%. (*4*) 8 nurses. (*5*) 120 ml. (*6*) 200 ml. (*7*) 66⅔%. (*8*) £21·13. (*9*) 340 adults. (*10*) £660 per annum.

Chapter 11, page 89

(*1*) 25 billion (25 million million). (*2*) 2500 sq m; 2916⅔ sq yd. (*3*) 60 cm³. (*4*) Neutrophils 40%, eosinophils 3⅓%, basophils 1⅔%, lymphocytes 43⅓%, monocytes 11⅔%. (*5*) 4,850,000 red cells per cu mm. (*6*) 5·9 g, 9·76 g, 11·8 g, 15·5 g.

Chapter 12, page 99

(*1*) 0·8 ml. (*2*) 0·8 ml. (*3*) 0·6 ml. (*4*) 0·75 ml. (*5*) 0·3 ml. (*6*) 0·6 ml. (*7*) 1·1 ml. (*8*) 0·75 ml.

page 101

(*1*) 1 in 40. (*2*) 1 in 5000. (*3*) 1 in 150. (*4*) 1 in 200.
(*5*) 1 in 200. (*6*) 1 in 250. (*7*) 1·25%. (*8*) 0·1%. (*9*) 2·5%.
(*10*) 1%. (*11*) 1 in 40. (*12*) 1 in 33⅓. (*13*) 1 in 25.
(*14*) 1 in 100. (*15*) 1 in 20. (*16*) (*a*) 2 ml, 1 in 50; (*b*) 4 oz, 10%;
(*c*) 300 ml, 1 in 100; (*d*) 1200 ml, 1¼%; (*e*) 640 ml, 1 in 160;
(*f*) 250 ml, 0·1%; (*g*) 3 ml, 1 in 10,000; (*h*) 8 ml, 1 in 5;
(*i*) 2 pints, 5%; (*j*) 3 ml, 1 in 40; (*k*) 10 ml, 1 in 200; (*l*) ½ oz, 1⅔%;
(*m*) 1 ml, 1 in 500; (*n*) 320 ml, 1 in 80; (*o*) 40 ml, 1¼%.

Chapter 13, page 110

(*1*) ⅓ ml. (*2*) 29·4 mg. (*3*) 0·15 mg. (*4*) 214 mg approximately.
(*5*) 590 mg. (*6*) 0·3 ml. (*7*) 12 mg. (*8*) 1·1 g.

page 110, problems

(*1*) Draw up ¾ of the Omnopon and discard the remainder.
(*2*) Take 6⅔ oz of the 1 in 20 strength and add 33⅓ oz of water.
(*3*) 3600 ml. (*4*) 625 ml. (*5*) 400 ml; 800 ml. (*6*) ⅝ (0·625) ml.
(*7*) 1⅓ ml. (*8*) Pethidine 75 mg; promethazine 37·5 mg. (*9*) 5 oz.
(*10*) Take 400 ml of 1 in 1000, add 200 ml water. (*11*) 75 ml of 1 in 5.
(*12*) 80 ml. (*13*) 1⅓ ml. (*14*) 2½ oz of 10%. (*15*) 900 ml.
(*16*) 20 ml. (*17*) 100 ml. (*18*) 4 litres, 750 ml. (*19*) 125 ml.
(*20*) 125 ml.

Chapter 14, page 122

(*3*) (*a*) 37·4°F; (*b*) 64·4°F; (*c*) 77·9°F; (*d*) 212°F; (*e*) 96·8°F;
(*f*) 107·6°F; (*g*) 122°F; (*h*) 158°F. (*4*) (*a*) 5°C; (*b*) 25°C;
(*c*) 13°C; (*d*) 40°C; (*e*) 30°C; (*f*) 26°C; (*g*) 185·5°C;
(*h*) 100°C. (*5*) (*a*) False; (*b*) true; (*c*) true; (*d*) true;
(*e*) false; (*f*) false; (*g*) false.

Chapter 15, page 135

(*1*) 2¼ hours. (*2*) 6 hours 21 minutes.

page 138

(*1*) 438·2 Calories. (*2*) 1624·4 Calories; 135·36 Calories.
(*3*) 58·2 Calories. (*4*) 78 Calories. (*5*) 280 ml milk.

Chapter 16, page 150

(*1*) Total force exerted = 4 tonnes, 200 kilograms. (*2*) ½ sq cm.
(*3*) 7·5 kg per sq cm, no. (*4*) 822 metres. (*5*) 107°C, the saline
will boil with explosive force. (*6*) 740 mm.

Chapter 17, page 162

(*1*) 140°F, 41°F, 68°F, 95°F, 151°F, 155°F, 167°F, 198°F.
(2) 10°C, 7°C, 22°C, 35½°C, 42°C, 52½°C, 59°C, 93°C, 37°C.

page 163

(*1*) No.   (2) 4·45 kg.   (3) 4½ weeks.   (4) No.   (5) Yes.
(*a*) 99·4°F = 37·5°C; 90;   (*b*) 102·6°F = 39·2°C; 122;   (*c*) 95;
(*d*) 100·5°F = 38·1°C   (6) (*a*) 22·1;   (*b*) 1·85;   (*c*) January;
(*d*) August.

Chapter 19, page 195

(*1*) (*a*) 54 = 110110;   (*b*) 47 = 101111;   (*c*) 23 = 10111;
(*d*) 35 = 100011;   (*e*) 143 = 10001111.
(2) (*a*) 27;   (*b*) 17;   (*c*) 53;   (*d*) 6;   (*e*) 341.
(*3*) (*a*) 10010010 = 146;   (*b*) 100000 = 32;   (*c*) 111100 = 60.
(*4*) (*a*) 10000 = 16;   (*b*) 1110 = 14;   (*c*) 10110 = 22.

NURSING BOOKS

NEW BOOKS AND NEW EDITIONS

VENEREAL DISEASES: TREATMENT AND NURSING
By H. Elliott S.R.N. and **K. Ryz** S.R.N., R.M.N., M.I.H.E.

Knowledge of the sexually transmitted diseases is now an important part of nurse training and this new book provides essential information on this subject. It covers the infection, diagnosis and treatment of syphilis, gonorrhoea, the nonspecific genital infections and other associated conditions. The authors write sympathetically about the situations the nurse will encounter, and their experience and understanding provide much valuable insight for the reader.
200 pages 16 illus 1 colour plate £1.80

PATIENT CARE: CARDIOVASCULAR DISORDERS
By Pat M. Ashworth S.R.N., S.C.M., and **Harry Rose** S.R.N., R.F.N., R.N.T., B.T.A.

This new textbook is designed for nurses who have completed some of their preliminary nursing studies and are ready to deepen their knowledge of the more specialized aspects of patient care. The authors have written a stimulating and very informative text which will be of value to both student and trained nurses.
240 pages 68 illus £2.80

NURSES' GUIDE TO CARDIAC MONITORING
By Peter Hubner M.B., B.S., M.R.C.P.

"This small book treats the whole subject of ECG monitoring in a very practical way, with clear examples of the traces as observed on the monitor . . . The value of this book is that it is short, concise and practical in its approach . . ." *Nursing Times 1971*
66 pages 35 illus £1.00

MAYES' MIDWIFERY: A TEXTBOOK FOR MIDWIVES
By Rosemary E. Bailey S.R.N., S.C.M., M.T.D., R.N.T., D.N.

This book has long been accepted as one of the classic textbooks for the midwife, and its clarity and completeness have been particularly welcomed by those studying for the examination of the Central Midwives Board. In this new eighth edition the text has been extensively rewritten and revised to take account of recent developments in obstetrics.
8th ed 530 pages 186 illus £2.50

BAILLIÈRE TINDALL 7 & 8 Henrietta Street
London WC2E 8QE

Reference Books

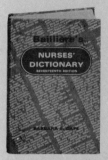

BAILLIÈRE'S NURSES' DICTIONARY
By Barbara F. Cape S.R.N., S.C.M., D.N.

"An informative, pocket-sized, nurses' dictionary
. . . low-price, compact book of reference can be
recommended to all, especially student and pupil
nurses at the start of their training."

Nursing Mirror 1969

| 17th ed | 572 pages | 8 plates | 50p |

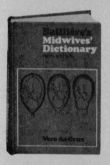

BAILLIÈRE'S MIDWIVES' DICTIONARY
By Vera Da Cruz S.R.N., S.C.M., M.T.D.

The ideal pocket-sized dictionary for midwives
and obstetric nurses. "A little mine of invaluable
information . . . it really does contain the exact
definition wanted in a hurry."

Midwives' Chronicle 1969

| 5th ed | 396 pages | 140 illus | 55p |

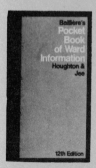

BAILLIÈRE'S POCKET BOOK OF WARD INFORMATION
By Marjorie Houghton
O.B.E., S.R.N., S.C.M., D.N.

and Ann Jee S.R.N., Part 1 C.M.B., R.N.T.

Fully revised and brought up-to-date, this book
contains a multitude of useful information likely
to be needed by nurses in their day to day work
and of particular help to nurses in training.

| 12th ed | 192 pages | 6 illus | 50p |

BAILLIÈRE TINDALL

7 & 8 Henrietta Street
London WC2E 8QE

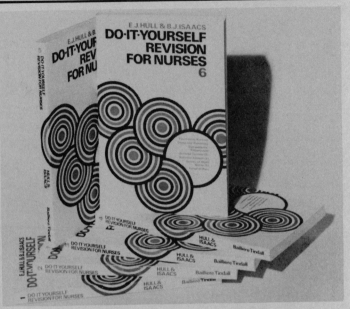

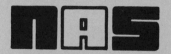 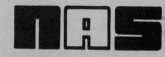
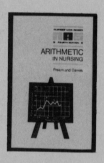
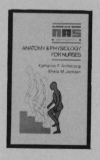
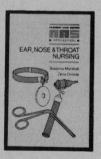

ANAESTHETICS FOR NURSES
by Joan Hobkirk S.R.N.
1st ed   90p

MEDICAL NURSING
by M. Houghton O.B.E.,
S.C.M., D.N., and C. M. Chapman
B.Sc.(Soc.), S.R.N.,
S.C.M., R.N.T.
8th ed   cloth £1.40 limp 90p

MICROBIOLOGY FOR NURSES
by E. J. Bocock and revised by
M. J. Parker, S.R.N.
4th ed   cloth £1.40 limp 90p

**OBSTETRIC AND
GYNAECOLOGICAL NURSING**
by R. E. Bailey S.R.N., S.C.M.,
M.T.D., R.N.T., D.N.
1st ed   cloth £1.40 limp 90p

ORTHOPAEDICS FOR NURSES
by W. Talog Davies and revised by
E. M. Stone, Hon. M.A.
S.R.N., S.C.M., R.N.T.
4th ed   cloth £1.40 limp 90p

PAEDIATRIC NURSING
by M. A. Duncombe S.R.N.,
R.S.C.N., S.C.M., and B. Weller
S.R.N., R.S.C.N., R.N.T.
3rd ed   cloth £1.20 limp 90p

**PERSONAL AND
COMMUNITY HEALTH**
by Winifred L. Huntly S.R.N.,
S.C.M., D.N.
2nd ed   cloth 80p limp 60p

PHARMACOLOGY FOR NURSES
by Rosemary E. Bailey S.R.N.,
S.T.D., D.N.
3rd ed   cloth £1.25 limp 90p

PRACTICAL NURSING
revised by M. Clarke B.Sc.,
S.R.N., R.N.T.
11th ed   cloth £1.40 limp 90p

PRACTICAL PROCEDURES
by M. Houghton O.B.E., S.R.N.,
S.C.M., D.N., and J. E. Parnell,
S.R.N., S.C.M., R.N.T.
1st ed   70p

PSYCHIATRIC NURSING
by A. Altschul B.A., S.R.N.,
R.M.N.
4th ed   cloth £1.50 limp £1.00

PSYCHOLOGY FOR NURSES
by A. Altschul B.A., S.R.N.,
R.M.N.
3rd ed   cloth £1.00 limp 90p

SURGICAL NURSING
by Katherine F. Armstrong and
revised by Peggy Sporne S.R.N.,
D.N., R.N.T.
8th ed   cloth £1.20 limp 90p

THEATRE TECHNIQUE
by Marjorie Houghton O.B.E.,
S.R.N., S.C.M., D.N., and
Jean Hudd, S.R.N.
4th ed   90p

**TROPICAL HYGIENE
AND NURSING**
by Wm. C. Fream S.R.N.,
B.T.A.Cert., S.T.D.
5th ed   90p

BAILLIÈRE TINDALL   7 & 8 Henrietta Street
                               London WC2E 8QE

: prices and details do not necessarily refer to current editions.

Standard Textbooks

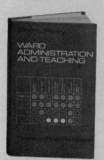

WARD ADMINISTRATION & TEACHING
By Ellen L. Perry

"This is a book which has long been needed. Every trained nurse could learn something from it. While ward sisters put into practice the ideals and ideas outlined, we need have no fears for 'patient care' in our hospitals nor for the practical training of the nurse." *Nursing Mirror*

304 pages   11 illus   £2.00

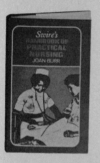

SWIRE'S HANDBOOK
OF PRACTICAL NURSING
Revised by Joan Burr R.M.N., S.R.N.

Changes in the syllabus of training have necessitated a major revision for this edition and Miss Burr has taken the opportunity to make many changes of approach to stress the human angle and to enable the nurse to appreciate her surroundings in the hospital and in the community. Care has been taken to cover the syllabus fully, and the use of simple language and illustrated examples ensure the maintained interest of the pupil.

6th ed   308 pages   57 illus   £1.10

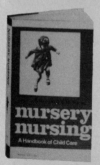

NURSERY NURSING—
A HANDBOOK FOR NURSERY NURSES
By A. B. Meering S.R.N., S.C.M.
and G. Stacey S.R.N.

"This book is written in a clear and simple style emphasizing the relationship between the emotional, intellectual and physical growth during infancy and childhood . . . a valuable reference book for all nurses interested in nursery work . . ." *The Lamp*

5th ed   414 pages   75 illus   £2.50

BAILLIÈRE TINDALL

7 & 8 Henrietta Street
London WC2E 8QE

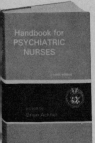

HANDBOOK FOR PSYCHIATRIC NURSES
Edited by the late Brian Ackner
M.D., F.R.C.P., D.P.M

"The R.M.P.A. is to be congratulated on sustaining its great tradition in nursing education by re-modelling its famous 'Handbook' to produce an entirely new account of psychiatry for nurses . . . this is an extremely readable and useful book."

Nursing Mirror

9th ed   364 pages   1 illus   £2.00

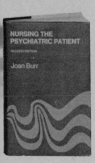

NURSING THE PSYCHIATRIC PATIENT
By Joan Burr R.M.N., S.R.N.

"This book has rapidly been acclaimed as an excellent addition to the psychiatric nursing textbooks already available, and it certainly provides a masterly account of what caring for the mentally ill is about . . . it is written with such sympathy that, should somebody recognise a description of their own difficulties, they could well gain comfort from the fact that such a helpful understanding is being disseminated."

Nursing Times reviewing the first edition

2nd ed   308 pages   10 illus   hard £1.50   limp £1.00

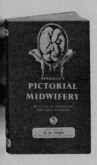

BERKELEY'S PICTORIAL MIDWIFERY
Revised by D. M. Stern
M.A., M.B., Ch.B., F.R.C.S., F.R.C.O.G.

A pictorial survey with excellent illustrations accompanied by clear descriptive text, which will prove invaluable to both the student and qualified midwife alike.

The book has a dual role, providing a text and atlas of theory and a reference for the practical aspects of the subject.

5th ed   176 pages   224 illus   2 coloured plates   £1.60

LLIÈRE TINDALL   7 & 8 Henrietta Street
London WC2E 8QE

REFERENCE AND SPECIALIST TEXTS

ATLAS OF FEMALE ANATOMY 7th ed
and ATLAS OF MALE ANATOMY 5th ed
By K. F. Armstrong S.R.N., S.C.M., D.N.(Lond.) & D. J. Kidd M.M.A.A.

To see is to learn! That is why these Atlases are so valuable, for they show clearly and accurately in colour and in black and white, the structure of the human body, giving the names of the various parts and outlining their functions in accompanying text. Separate cut-out pictures of each organ are provided for positioning on the atlas diagrams. Great attention has been paid to accuracy of detail even in the smallest illustrations, with a key index naming every part and a clear and concise explanatory text.

Female Atlas 17" x 9¼" 32 pages 5 colour plates £1.60
Male Atlas 17" x 9¼" 34 pages 4 colour, 3 black and white plates £1.60

NURSING CARE OF THE UNCONSCIOUS PATIENT
By P. Mountjoy S.R.N., R.M.N., and B. Wythe S.R.N., R.M.N.

"This book should be in the hands of all doctors as well as medical students and nurses who have the care of such patients. As head injuries are the modern plague and all hospitals have these patients then no one can go wrong who follows this guide. It is almost made too easy but this problem is not as difficult as is sometimes alleged but it is a matter of getting things right from the start. We know of no guiding light that is quite as good as this book." *New Zealand Medical Journal*

97 pages 11 illus 90p

AN INSIGHT INTO HEALTH VISITING
By Mary K. Chisholm R.G.N., S.C.M., H.V.(Cert.)

"Very rarely have I enjoyed reading a textbook so much. Intended as an introduction to health visiting for student nurses, it presents a most attractive job with plenty of work satisfaction.

It is well written, easily read and should maintain the interest of the student nurse as it is related throughout to her present knowledge within the hospital walls and is copiously illustrated with appropriate anecdotes. Miss Chisholm is to be congratulated on presenting the health visitor's work and value to the community in such a lucid and attractive manner." *District Nursing*

102 pages 60p

BAILLIÈRE TINDALL ⚜

7 & 8 Henrietta Street
London WC2E 8QE

The prices and details quoted in this list are those current at the time of going to press but are liable to subsequent alteration without notice and local currency fluctuations.
Printed in Great Britain 2/73